The 50+ Plan

His and Hers HRT

Dr Malcolm Carruthers

D1350522

Clink Street

London | New York

Published by Clink Street Publishing 2017

Copyright © 2017

First edition.

The author asserts the moral right under the Copyright, Designs and Patents Act 1988 to be identified as the author of this work.

All rights reserved. No part of this publication may be reproduced, stored in a retrieval system or transmitted, in any form or by any means without the prior consent of the author, nor be otherwise circulated in any form of binding or cover other than that with which it is published and without a similar condition being imposed on the subsequent purchaser.

ISBNs: 978-1-912262-94-6 paperback, 978-1-912262-75-5 ebook

Disclaimer

This book has been written purely from the belief that millions of men and women worldwide are being denied the many benefits of hormonal treatments because of the multiple influences discussed in this book. No, I am not in the pay of that popular ogre 'Big Pharma' or funded by other commercial organisations.

I am medical consultant to the Centre for Men's Health, a company running clinics in London's Harley Street, and Manchester, but do not have shares in it. I am still in clinical practice part-time but am not financially dependent on it

The ideas and suggestions in this book are based on the clinical experience and medical training of the author and scientific articles available. Every attempt has been made to present current and accurate information as of time of publication. The suggestions in this book are definitely not meant to be a substitute for careful medical evaluation and treatment by a qualified, licensed health professional. Each person's health need's, risks, and goals are different and should be developed with medical supervision for personalized advice, answers to specific medical questions, and individual recommendations. The author and publisher specifically do not recommend starting any new treatment, changing any medication you may be taking, or using over-the-counter hormone preparations without consulting your personal physician. This book is intended for educational purposes only, and use of the information is intended for educational purposes only, and use of the information is entirely at the reader's discretion. The author and publisher cannot be responsible for any adverse reactions arising directly or indirectly from the suggestions in this material, and specifically disclaim any liability from the use of this book.

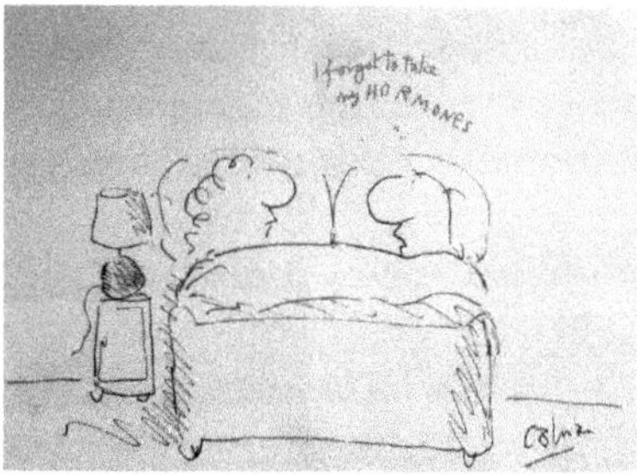
I forgot to take
my HORMONES

To patients who have taught me so much about the benefits of testosterone treatment and HRT for their partners together with friends and colleagues who have supported me in the fight for testosterone replacement treatment (TRT), especially Mark Feneley, Professor Tom Trinick, Dr Adrian Zentner, Professor Ralph Martins, Professor Bruno Lunenfeld, Professor Svetlana Kalinchenko, Professor Abe Morgentaler, and many others round the world. My sons, Andrew and Robert, also had valuable comments on the manuscript.

A special thank you to Dr Lee Vliet who contributed a lot of her wisdom and experience to the book.

Last but not least, to my wife, Jean Coleman, Secretary and Cofounder of the Andropause Society, who has constantly supported me over the last thirty years and helped me sustain and survive the fight for the male hormone.

Contents

The Fifty-Plus Plan – His and Hers HRT:

A basis for medical care after fifty for both men and women

Introduction

With advances in medical science, and a lot of luck, you may well live to be 100. The only remaining question is 'How enjoyable and healthy can you make the second half of your life?' This is the question this book sets out to answer.

Around the age of fifty, women go through a hormonal crisis usually called the menopause, and at a more variable age in men, the less recognized andropause. In women, this is jokingly referred to as the work of the seven dwarves: itchy, bitchy, sweaty, bloaty, sleepy, forgetful and psycho. These symptoms are common and distressing. They are caused by the ovaries slowing down or stopping production of estrogens as they run out of ovarian follicles.

Apart from the loss of periods, there are emotional changes which include increased irritability, and a fluctuating depression. Women going through this often object to just two things about their partners – everything they say and everything they do. There may also be joint stiffness and loss of skin elasticity. Osteoporosis may result in gradually reducing stature and even accidental fractures, particularly of the hips, though fortunately these do not occur till the sixties and seventies or later.

With men, the reduction of testosterone activity is usually more gradual, but the symptoms can be just as severe.

Instead of losing their periods, they usually experience difficulty in getting and maintaining an erection. The most characteristic warning sign is losing their morning erections, the 'morning glories', which is due to a reduction in testosterone activity. This can be considered as the male equivalent of the loss of periods in women.

Again they can experience remarkably similar physical and mental symptoms to menopausal women including irritability, depression, inability to concentrate, joint pains and even hot flushes.

These symptoms in both sexes can severely reduce enjoyment of life and love, and even cause relationships to break down both at home and at work.

The question should be asked 'why put up with them?' when HRT can prevent and generally even reverse them safely and effectively, and stop associated illnesses developing. It's what most people would call a no-brainer, but it is still not accepted by many doctors. This book makes the case, which I believe is an important one for the future health of an aging population.

It's our sex hormones, estrogens in women and testosterone in men, that let us down, and even though the pattern of hormonal ageing is different in the two sexes a crisis point is often reached around the age of fifty in both. The fall in estrogen is often rapid in women, with dramatic onset of symptoms, loss of periods, hot flushes and night sweats.

Even so, a British Menopause Society Survey in 2016 showed that despite the symptoms having a significant adverse effect on the quality of their lives, only half of the women consulted their doctors to try to get any help. Such is the low expectation of any positive advice or help being available (see Figure 1).

Figure 1

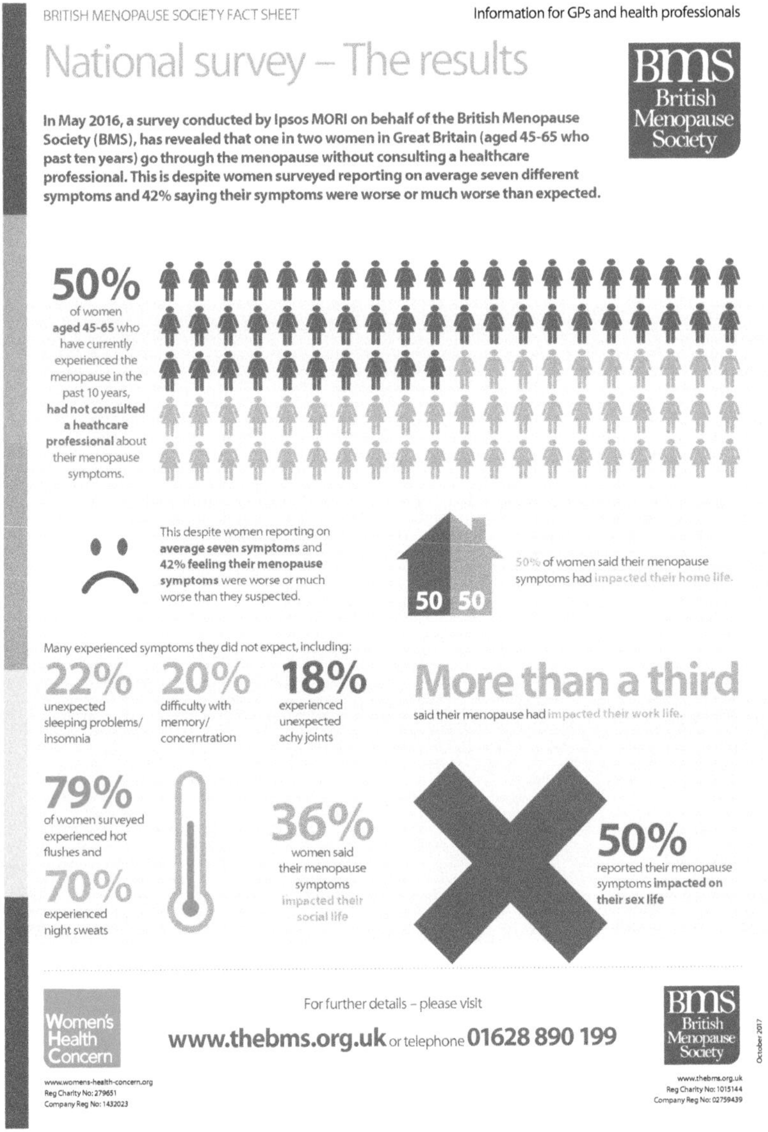
BRITISH MENOPAUSE SOCIETY FACT SHEET
Information for GPs and health professionals
National survey – The results
BMS British Menopause Society
In May 2016, a survey conducted by Ipsos MORI on behalf of the British Menopause Society (BMS), has revealed that one in two women in Great Britain (aged 45-65 who past ten years) go through the menopause without consulting a healthcare professional. This is despite women surveyed reporting on average seven different symptoms and 42% saying their symptoms were worse or much worse than expected.
50% of women aged 45-65 who have currently experienced the menopause in the past 10 years, had not consulted a heathcare professional about their menopause symptoms.
This despite women reporting on average seven symptoms and 42% feeling their menopause symptoms were worse or much worse than they suspected.
50 50
50% of women said their menopause symptoms had impacted their home life.
Many experienced symptoms they did not expect, including:
22% unexpected sleeping problems/ insomnia
20% difficulty with memory/ concerntration
18% experienced unexpected achy joints
More than a third said their menopause had impacted their work life.
79% of women surveyed experienced hot flushes and
70% experienced night sweats
36% women said their menopause symptoms impacted their social life
50% reported their menopause symptoms impacted on their sex life
Women's Health Concern
www.womens-health-concern.org
Reg Charity No: 279651
Company Reg No: 1432023
For further details – please visit
www.thebms.org.uk or telephone 01628 890 199
BMS British Menopause Society
www.thebms.org.uk
Reg Charity No: 1015144
Company Reg No: 02759439
October 2017

This is in spite of a recommendation by NICE (National Institute for Clinical Excellence in the UK) in November 2015 which was generally very supportive of using HRT if the woman wished it. Few general practitioners are encouraging, or willing to undertake the responsibility of starting a woman on HRT.

This is in contrast to the cosmetics industry, which is spending vast amounts of money on marketing anti-ageing creams of largely unproven effectiveness. However, this is non-controversial as the women pay for this themselves, and the treatment has a strong placebo effect.

Everyone knows the symptoms of the menopause and what it represents. It is the time in a woman's life when about the age of fifty, her ovaries begin to run out of the ovarian follicles which produce the estrogen hormone that makes her fertile and gives her monthly periods.

This hormonal reduction is accompanied by symptoms which range from mild to life- and relationship-wrecking. A survey by the British Menopause Society in 2016 showed the results on the next page (Figure 1). As you can see, they often include loss of energy and libido, depression, insomnia and night sweats and hot flushes, causing her to refrigerate both the bedroom and her partner. There may be joint pains and stiffness, lethargy and loss of figure in spite of exercise, together with weight gain.

What can make this series of changes in her life worse is that her husband of about the same age may be suffering remarkably similar symptoms, often laughingly referred to as the 'male menopause'. As well as loss of energy and libido, his get up and go has often got up and gone, and action man becomes inaction man, often experiencing erratic erections, with the most characteristic sign being loss of early morning erections, sometimes called morning glories.

After a restless night sleep for both partners, he may resemble a depressed irritable bear with a sore head. This combination of his and hers symptoms is a great strain on any relationship. This is illustrated by the following case histories of a husband and wife team up in the north of Scotland, showing the difference that TRT and HRT can make to his and her health.

Ian's story

For the first time in my life, when I reached my late fifties I started to suffer from all manner of symptoms of joint pains and loss of energy. I had always been the boss during my working life, carrying all responsibilities and pressures without any problem. Very quickly this situation got worse and I found myself developing a ferocious temper for no apparent reason and began to suffer from severe night sweats as well as a feeling that the entire world was conspiring to work against me. After a very thorough wide range of tests at the local teaching hospital I was told that I was very fit for my age but had to realise that I was getting older and this natural deterioration was causing my depression. I was offered Prozac to reduce my stress levels but I told them where to put it, as I was sure that there was another deeper factor causing my problems.

By chance I heard of Dr Malcolm Carruthers and his work with TRT in ageing males. I arranged to go to London and be examined by him. After a very thorough medical and wide range of lab tests he told me that I was suffering from a very low free available testosterone level and assured me that with a suitable TRT treatment I would be back to my normal vigorous self in a relatively short time. This was in February 1997, when Dr Carruthers also told me I was the physically fittest sixty-year-old male he had ever encountered.

I was prescribed Restandol tablets at that time for my treatment and within a few days felt as if I was reborn. I continued to be treated with these hormone capsules for several years but in time became more aware that variations in my diet causing poor absorption of the capsules appeared to reduce their effects.

Dr Carruthers then recommended TRT implants for me. These provided the necessary TRT but it was found that my body unfortunately always rejected and expelled the medication pellets long before their proscribed implantation period was ever reached.

By this time the Australian Andromen TRT cream became available and I was using this product very satisfactorily for some time.

Then, in 2007, Tostran 2% Gel became available and I have been using this medication ever since. It is easily applied, accurately measured and of a relatively low cost. I am now 80 years old, still very fit and with a high libido and enjoying life to the full in every respect.

I believe that my long term use of TRT is entirely responsible for this extended length and quality of my life. Particularly when I remember that I had reached the point of almost being suicidal when I started my continuous prescribed TRT medication, now over twenty years ago.

Lillian's Story – coming alive at sixty-five

Early every morning my husband reaches out for me and in next to no time I am transported to a plateau of wonderful sexual excitement and pleasure.

These feelings are way beyond anything that I was capable of experiencing during the first forty years of our marriage.

I used to say that my 'internal wiring' was incomplete or nonexistent, and that I was 'dead' inside. But – that is not the case now!

Hubby always wanted to give me feelings of pleasure that I was not capable of achieving. Physical pleasure for me did not develop to any great degree. Instead, love-making would become wearing and I could be close to tears and would want to abandon it. Even after a time apart when I would be longing to be in hubby's arms, physical excitement did not develop as it should. Sharing stimulating literature provided mental stimulation which failed to develop into physical excitement.

Was my upbringing preventing me from having a fulfilling sexual relationship? No. I was married and I had no doubt that sex was a vital part of our relationship.

Was it fear of pregnancy? Possibly, or so I thought. When our family was complete and the possibility of pregnancy was terminated there was still no improvement. Hubby thought that it must be his fault and that he should be able to bring about responses in me that were not materialising. As I approached retirement and would not be expending energy at work, I hoped that I might be able to achieve more sexual pleasure. Of course, this was just more wishful thinking.

Five years ago, having learnt about the existence of post menopausal HRT and its benefits, I consulted my GP and he started me on Livial, which has a small testosterone-like action. When I had been on Livial for only a few weeks I began to see improvement in my skin texture, my hair and muscle tone. I also began to get pleasure from my breasts/nipples being caressed, and long periods of continuous excitement. This extended stimulation and pleasure resulted in my vagina becoming aroused and increasingly well lubricated. (My internal wiring was coming alive.)

My husband had attended the Men's Health Clinic in Harley Street and through Dr Carruthers learned that in

Australia there were Women Too clinics where women are also treated with testosterone. After conducting an internet search we discovered that many couples had been helped and were benefiting from this treatment. We found that Androfem cream was available online. Three years ago I started to apply a tiny spot of cream daily onto the clitoris hood and surrounding area. Soon the clitoris became much enlarged and much more sensitive, and when stimulated sexual lubrication increased dramatically as well. Around the same time I realised that some hair was growing on my chin. There was also a slight increase of hair growth on my lower tummy and tops of my thighs. This problem was completely manageable, however. Hubby remembers that for a time my tummy used to swell a bit during sexual arousal. I am about five pounds heavier, but no one would notice as it does not show. My tummy is less flabby now and I have not grown out of any clothes.

For some time now very exciting things have been happening inside me. Although all my orgasms up till now have been clitoral orgasms, my internal areas and particularly my G spot have become very responsive and we believe that one day soon I might even experience a full internal orgasm. The internal areas behind the G spot are awake and working really well. My husband must have thought that the awakening was complete when the head/neck of my cervix started to pump to meet his penis. Another surprise was occasional spontaneous spurting during height of arousal.

All the advice and techniques we took on board in the past trying to get satisfaction work wonders for us now, because of the change in me brought about by the daily application of a tiny spot of cream. I am sure now that my 'internal wiring' was always complete, only my testosterone level could not quite get the current to flow. We can now enjoy giving each other unlimited sexual pleasures as we approach our seventies.

Better late than never, but had the opportunity to have this small adjustment to my hormone balance been available twenty years ago, would I have been spared monthly migraines, prolonged PMT, tender breasts, lack of benefit from sleep, low mental and physical energy levels, and painful knee joints? At that time I operated like a robot with flat batteries with absolutely NO physical response to lovemaking.

My husband happened to see on TV a documentary in which the benefits of HRT were explained. I then went to see my GP and he agreed to start me on HRT. The migraines stopped and I felt unwell for only one day a month. Life improved greatly. I was no longer so tired that I was miserable. I got back to what had been my best.

I was born too soon for the 'Women Too' clinics, and in the wrong country. I am glad for those Australian women who are like I was but have access to those clinics.

I am so thankful that we came across the HRT information and decided to use it. It has helped various aspects of my person. I am now calmer and more confident. I feel fitter than ever, have no aches or pains, and at last can reward my husband with encouraging responses that he had long since given up hoping for.

Why do women and their partners put up with these symptoms and serious interference with the quality of their lives without seeking help?

Unfortunately, with increasing pressure on the health services in most countries as populations age, it is difficult for either partner to get reliable, sympathetic, knowledgeable advice from a general physician. Often the woman is told 'This is just your age – It's the change – It's perfectly natural – Come back in a year or two and we will consider whether you need treatment for it – What? You are about to lose your husband and your job? Ah, well I can give you antidepressants or sleeping pills or refer you for psychotherapy or couples' counselling. No, I don't want to discuss HRT until you have tried "natural remedies" for a year or two.'

Hormones are like the water that a plant needs to keep it healthy or even alive. Would you deprive a plant of it till it wilts, and then try and revive it by belatedly drenching it, and being surprised when it stays wilted?

This attitude of many doctors is due to a mixture of reasons which will be discussed in the next chapter under the heading 'hormonophobia', a common medical affliction, the reasons for which will be explained later.

Because of the common failure to recognize these symptoms in the male, the diagnosis is seldom made, and the hormone deficiencies of estrogen in the woman and testosterone in the man go untreated for 2–5 years until lasting damage has been done to health, the relationship or both. Also, many studies have shown that HRT is safest if started as soon as the initial symptoms appear.

It has been widely accepted by the medical profession and the general public alike that women may choose to spend much of their reproductive lives, ages 18–45, on oral contraceptives usually containing various mixtures of estrogen and progesterone. It may be claimed that a few women's lives are lost by complications such as thromboembolism, but this has to be weighed against sexual pleasure and freedom to choose your partner and prevent deaths and sterility from septic abortions and unwanted pregnancies. Aside from religious objections, I believe it is the woman's right to choose. Why not extend the carefully monitored use of these hormones into later life to prolong mental and physical well-being?

This book is offered in an attempt to overcome these

objections to 'His and Hers HRT', and make them a basis for maintaining good health in both partners for as long as possible as they travel through the second half of their lives.

With the help of hormones they can live their lives in square wave form, like alkaline batteries going full charge to the end!

Chapter 1 - Hormonophobia

This is the largely irrational fear that many doctors have, and pass on to their patients, of using hormones such as estrogen and testosterone to prolong active life by preventing or treating the miseries and illnesses that deficiencies of these hormones can cause in the second half of life. It is, as I see it, denying the doctor's basic duty 'to comfort always'. Take your pick:

1. Failure to realise the urgency of the situation. Not understanding the severe impact that the combined symptomatology can have on the quality of life, and the associated disease processes which may be starting due to hormone deficiencies.
2. Medical orthodoxy
3. Lack of a true understanding of the safety of an increasing range of TRT and HRT preparations
4. Fears which have been generated by previous studies
5. Fears about the cost/benefits of different forms of TRT and HRT
6. Unwillingness to take responsibility for putting a man or woman on hormonal treatment and keeping them on it for several years or even, using it as part of the basis of a health-promoting regime, for life, as this book recommends.

The fate of the man who plucks up his courage to complain to his doctor of his menopause-like symptoms, or is urged by his partner to do so, is even harder. He is told he is just depressed, and treated with antidepressants, or given Viagra for his erection problems, which only works temporarily or not all, and doesn't solve the other emotional or physical symptoms.

If he persists in thinking that his symptoms may be caused by low testosterone he is given a blood test which routinely shows that his level is 'within the normal range' so he can't have low-T, can he? Unfortunately, this doesn't rule out 'Low T-Activity', due to testosterone resistance, similar to the low insulin activity seen in diabetics due to insulin resistance, which only recognition of the typical symptoms and a trial of testosterone treatment will establish.

Factors contributing to this medical inactivity are:

1. Failure to realize the urgency of the situation

The symptoms of estrogen deficiency in menopausal women, especially the sexual symptoms of lack of libido and reduced enjoyment of intercourse, together with irritability and impaired memory, can cause friction in relationships and trouble at work. This can lead to divorce and loss of employment.

Similarly I have seen many men with marital problems due to the depression, and irritability, resulting in low libido and erection problems caused by testosterone deficiency. Loss of drive and reduced efficiency at work, together with irritability, are common and may lead to loss of income and redundancy. Also, as will be described later, a wide range of illnesses ranging from heart disease to diabetes can start up in the early years of these low hormone activity states, complications routinely ignored at the patient's peril.

2. Medical Orthodoxy

This has its roots deep in medical training. With the motto 'Firstly, do no harm' and a five- or six-year training program before they are let loose to the public, as well as another five- or six-year postgraduate program before they are expected to practise as independent specialists, it is unsurprising that doctors seldom think for themselves. Instead, their thoughts and deeds tend to be prescribed for them by their peers and seniors, often in the form of consensus and guidelines. These are sent down as from oracular beings, usually in the form of peer-reviewed articles in leading journals.

You can tell it is a leading journal by its 'impact factor', which ranges from the top holy writ of the *New England Journal of Medicine* at 50 in general medicine to the other American heavyweight *Journal of the American Medical Association* at 30, with most specialist journals weighing in at a puny 3–4. In the UK, as in America, there are two big ones, *The Lancet* at 39, and the *British Medical Journal* at only 16.

Also, these journals like to blow their own trumpets and make headlines in the newspapers and media by having well-oiled publicity machines to announce their latest papers to both doctors and the general public. These pronouncements are amplified by the relevant pharmaceutical companies if they are favourable and are played down by hired guns of experts with opposing views if they are unfavourable. This can and does lead to a bias toward eminence-based medicine rather than evidence-based medicine.

As for the young researcher, it is a question of publish

or perish, and your next research grant may depend on singing a popular song, while thinking outside the box is not encouraged. This can endanger your career, your job prospects, and your research grants. It might even get you struck off the medical register and stopped from practising if your ideas are sufficiently unorthodox and heretical. This is the equivalent of being excommunicated from the church if you are judged a radical priest. It forms a strong tide of medical opinion if you choose to swim against it.

Another impediment to a balanced evaluation of the literature is that these leading journals usually don't provide abstracts on any of the search databases, so that the pronouncements only come down from the Olympic heights of academia translated by medical journalists or press releases to newspapers. This results in extensive filtering of messages and considerable difficulty and expense if you wish to analyze the original paper.

3. Lack of awareness of newer, safer preparations

Often it is not realized by either doctors or their patients that certain preparations are intrinsically safe, especially in low doses. Often these forms of the hormone are the same molecules as occur naturally in the human body, so-called 'bio-identical' forms. While not believing that there is any particular magic in these forms, study after study has shown that the body seems better able to process these naturally occurring forms of the hormones rather than synthetic ones or those from other species.

A classical example of this is the relative safety of human estrogen in HRT formulations compared to equine estrogens from the urine of pregnant mares, a different molecule with important safety differences and actions. Also, to prevent overgrowth of the lining of the uterus due to using estrogen alone, in HRT preparations it is often combined with progesterone. Again, a natural form of progesterone appears relatively safe as compared to any of the synthetic forms of 'progestogen', an artificially synthesized form of molecule which is foreign to the human body and more likely to be toxic as shown in study after study.

Unfortunately these artificial forms of the hormones are often cheaper to manufacture, easier to patent, and designed to be better absorbed, which make them more attractive to and profitable to market than the natural hormones.

Another example of this is the synthetic hormone methyl testosterone, which had the advantages of being cheap and orally active, and came on the market in the mid-1930s and for a time became quite popular as a male form of TRT. Though only differing from testosterone by one chemical group, it was more easily converted to estrogen, and was toxic to the heart and liver, even causing cancer. However, because it was cheap it remained quite popular in many countries until the end of the last century, especially in Russia, and has only recently been taken off the market in Canada.

4. Fears which have been generated by previous studies

The big one here is the Women's Health Initiative (WHI) published in 2002. It was started in 1991 by the National Institute of Health in the USA, and was the largest and most expensive clinical research ever conducted into women's health. It involved over 16,000 women, mainly in their sixties and seventies, who had an intact uterus and another 10,000 hysterectomised group. The first received Premarin (equine estrogen), though it had long been regarded as the least-favourable form of HRT, plus

Provera (medroxyprogesterone acetate), a cheap and patented derivative of natural progesterone. This combination was the cheapest and most commonly used form of HRT in America, and made a huge study possible. The second group received Premarin only or a placebo.

One interesting fact about equine estrogen which was known even before the WHI study started is that unlike other natural estrogens, it actually reduced the amount of free estrogens and testosterone in the blood by increasing the binding protein, hormone-binding globulin. But that unintended consequence didn't stop the wrong preparations from being used.

So here we had two artificial compounds, neither of which was native to the human body, being used in women who were also generally outside the optimal age to start HRT, the window of opportunity for maximum safety and effectiveness. A badly designed experiment on thousands of women giving predictably bad results.

When it was time to publish the results the writing group, in what has since been described as an 'extraordinary decision' in a recently published book *Managing the Menopause*, released their results to health reporters on 10 July 2002, one week prior to the publication of the evidence in *JAMA*. This tactic appeared designed to induce maximum fear and confusion before the general medical profession had a chance to review the evidence.

Also, it seemed that the results had been reported in relative values rather than absolute values as a deliberate attempt to magnify the adverse events and strike fear into the minds of women and their clinicians using HRT. In this it succeeded brilliantly, and the majority of women on HRT worldwide came off it on what, when properly analyzed, was insufficient evidence.

The long-term finding was that after eleven years and much misery from withdrawal, the risk of stroke was not increased, the risk of deep vein thrombosis was decreased, and the risk of breast cancer was reduced by 23 percent. Also, the risk of hip fracture was increased by 55 percent when a woman stopped her HRT, but still, many doctors turned their minds and opinions against HRT, choosing the always attractive do-nothing option, and strongly advised against it. Neither was the marriage breakdown rate recorded in the untreated group. What an expensive public health disaster! Yet still, the misreported findings of the WHI study are also routinely used as evidence against any enthusiasm expressed for either HRT or, worse still, TRT.

5. Objections on grounds of costs

Faced with the greater use of hormonal preparations to stem the tide of diseases of ageing, health authorities claim it would be unaffordable. No it isn't, actually, being no more expensive than simple medications used to treat the conditions it prevents such as heart disease, depression and osteoporosis. Using a range of arguments, legislators look around for ways to make savings by cutting back on the drugs bill, especially where a group of doctors can be found to say it is an unnecessary expense.

It then becomes a case of considering the costs versus benefits of preventive medicine, especially if someone wants to invest a reasonable amount of their own money in taking the chance of prolonging their healthy active later lifespan. It could be compared to preventing a car breaking down by getting it regularly serviced.

Fortunately, cost-benefit analyses have already been carried out in Scandinavia and America by doctors making the case for HRT for men. The first was Professor Stefan

Arver, an endocrinologist in the Karolinska University in Stockholm. The aim of this analysis was to evaluate health outcomes and costs associated with lifelong TRT in patients suffering from testosterone deficiency.

Using a clever decision programme for patients being at continuous risk of disease events, called a Markov model, his team assessed the cost-effectiveness of testosterone undecanoate (TU) depot injection treatment compared with no treatment. Health outcomes and associated costs were modeled in monthly cycles per patient individually along a lifetime horizon. Modeled health outcomes included development of type 2 diabetes, depression, cardiovascular and cerebrovascular complications, and fractures.

The main outcome measures were quality-adjusted life years (QALYs) and total cost in TU depot injection treatment and no treatment cohorts. In addition, outcomes were also expressed as incremental cost per QALY gained for TU depot injection therapy compared with no treatment (incremental cost-effectiveness ratio (ICER)).

Outcomes in the testosterone deficient population estimated benefits of TRT at twenty euros (twenty-five USD) per QALY gained. Improvement in the reduced risk of developing type 2 diabetes had the highest impact on long-term outcomes.

This analysis suggests that lifelong TU depot injection therapy of patients with testosterone deficiency is a cost-effective treatment in Sweden and that there is a strong case for doing so, though this has largely been ignored by the authorities. This conclusion is obtained with treatment using injected testosterone and can be even more effective if the cheapest form of treatment with a gel applied to the scrotum, at a third of the cost, had been used.

A similar study in America at Baylor College, Houston, also in 2013, modeled the costs associated with testosterone-related complications, including cardiovascular disease (CVD), diabetes mellitus (DM), and osteoporosis-related fractures (ORFs). Incidence, prevalence, and mortality of these conditions were collected for men aged forty-five to seventy-four from six national databases and large cross-sectional studies. Relative risk (RR) rates were determined for these events in patients with testosterone less than 300 ng/dL (10nmol/L). The prevalence of testosterone deficiency was determined for this cohort of men.

Actual and adjusted (normalized for T deficiency) rates of CVD, DM, and ORFs in US men aged forty-five to seventy-four assuming a TD prevalence of 13.4 percent were calculated. It was determined that, over a twenty-year period, T deficiency is projected to be involved in the development of approximately 1.3 million new cases of CVD, 1.1 million new cases of DM, and over 600,000 ORFs. In year 1, the attributed cost burden of these diseases was approximately $8.4 billion.

It was calculated that over the entire twenty-year period, T deficiency may be directly responsible for approximately $190–$525 billion in inflation-adjusted US health-care expenditures. It was concluded that testosterone deficiency may be a significant contributor to adverse public health and that further study is needed to definitively describe whether testosterone deficiency is a modifiable risk factor for the diseases studied. This may represent an opportunity for nationwide public health initiatives aimed at preventive care.

Despite these carefully quantified financial studies on both sides of the Atlantic on the impact of testosterone deficiency on men's health in financial terms, there still seems remarkably little political will to make testosterone treatment available, even in limited areas, to see what such an experiment in preventive medicine can actually achieve. This may be because politicians are interested in quick fixes rather than immediate expenditure, whose benefits may not be apparent until after the next election in a few years' time. This is known as a limited-event horizon, which dictates much of medical policy.

6. Unwillingness to take responsibility for putting a woman on HRT, and keeping her on it for several years or even, using it a part of the basis of a health promoting regime, for life, as this book recommends

Both HRT and TRT need to be started and then supervised by doctors. This involves the patient starting up a long-term relationship, with the medical services taking some long-term responsibility for supervising the treatment.

Unfortunately, over the age of fifty, the frequency of most diseases, whether it's heart or circulatory disease, various forms of cancer or even dementia, rise.

Generally, the longer you live, the more prone to illness you are, and it has to be faced that the mortality of life is 100%. It's the quality of your life as well as your longevity that you want to maximize.

When men or women, having discussed the pros and cons, start on any form of hormonal treatment, any illness that follows even ten, twenty or thirty years later they might attribute to the hormones, even if there is no proven link – so-called ad hoc reasoning. If doctors encourage any form of preventive medication, and any illness occurs, when answering the eternal question 'Why me O lord?' the patient may come up with the answer 'It must be the hormone treatment!'

All products are tried and tested before they go on the market and the ones found to significantly increase the risk of any disease are continuously being weeded out during post-marketing surveillance and in the light of further clinical evidence.

It's like investing in the stock market. You take the advice of the best broker (doctor) you can find, take his advice and then act accordingly, with modern, safe preparations and continuous monitoring of the investment in your health account (shares). As with other investments, however, nothing is guaranteed, and you may take a 'health hit'. However with careful monitoring, any problems which arise should be detected early either by symptoms or six-monthly or yearly health checks, and corrected.

This is the philosophy behind the Fifty-Plus Plan for men and women, which will be explained in detail in the final chapter.

Chapter 2 – HRT for Men

There is a backlash against testosterone treatment by the medical establishment and allied forces, which can be called external resistance, as well as the original idea presented previously of internal resistance to the hormone in the body. This unrecognized factor is similar to the insulin resistance which is accepted as being the major cause of adult diabetes.

The argument of the external resistance forces goes: Because of heavy marketing by pharmaceutical companies that make testosterone preparations, sales, which were stable for years, have risen more than 1,800 percent in the United States, exceeding $1.9 billion in 2012. If, like most authorities, you define *testosterone deficiency* as a blood level below a certain value, then the frequency of the condition has not changed much over that period. There you are, they say, and defined this way the increased sales of the hormone are due to marketing hype and disease-mongering, and it is medically unnecessary, dangerous, and must be curtailed.

However, if you define it as a set of symptoms which gives you an identikit picture of the condition, then the number of patients who are aware of the disorder and try, usually without success, to convince their doctors to give them a trial of testosterone treatment, has increased by that amount or more. These symptoms include loss of libido, erection problems (particularly loss of morning erections), loss of energy, feeling of suddenly growing old, memory loss, depression, irritability, joint pains, and night sweats (See Ageing Male Symptoms questionnaire at end of book). They have been recognized as being associated with insufficient testosterone for over seventy years and are now being linked to several serious and increasingly common medical conditions such as diabetes and obesity.

If these characteristic symptoms then go away and stay away with a course of testosterone treatment and return when it's stopped, it is not just ageing, and patients naturally want to stay on the treatment.

However, lab-test-obsessed doctors will demand low testosterone levels as well even if, as shown in many research studies, including my own practical experience in treating more than 2,500 patients over twenty-five years, these levels bear no relation to the symptoms except when they are very low. This simple but effective approach is on the basis of the old saying that 'if it looks like a duck, walks like a duck, and quacks like a duck, it's a duck'.

The medical resistance movement is led by the endocrinologists, who regard themselves as the high priests of modern, lab-centred medicine. They overlook the crucial principle of testosterone resistance in the body. This is strange as many of these specialists also treat patients with diabetes, which in the majority of cases, as has been established for over seventy years, is due to resistance to the hormone insulin. If this key cause of diabetes had not been accepted by doctors fifty years ago before insulin could be measured but instead had been found to be high, according to the same logic, the hormone would have been denied to many patients to this day with disastrous consequences.

The fact remains that of the more than 20 percent of men over the age of fifty with symptoms of testosterone deficiency, only 1 percent are getting testosterone treatment in the UK and even less throughout Europe. America is doing better, and due to demand and advertising, is up nearer the 10 percent mark for men over fifty.

If this were thyroid-hormone deficiency and treatment rates, there would be a national and international outcry in deprived countries. But because of what I call testosterone resistance among medical professionals, deficiency of this hormone goes unrecognized and untreated, like the proverbial elephant in the doctor's consulting room. Let's see why this is and how we can do better.

Why Is Testosterone Deficiency Syndrome so Seldom Diagnosed or Treated?

As is usual, a *syndrome* in medicine can be defined as the association of several clinically recognizable features, including both signs and symptoms. It is derived from the Greek word συνδρομή (*sundromē*) and means 'concurrence of symptoms'.

Certainly, testosterone deficiency conforms to the definition of a syndrome because whatever its cause, whether sudden castration, anti-androgen drugs, or simply ageing, the constellation of symptoms produced is highly characteristic, specific, and can usually be relieved by a therapeutic trial of testosterone replacement therapy (TRT). The typical identikit pattern of symptoms includes loss of energy, drive, and libido, erectile dysfunction, memory loss, irritability, and depression and is sometimes accompanied by night sweats and hot flushes.

The peak age of onset is around fifty. The similarity to the female menopause and its symptoms is striking and has resulted in it being called the male climacteric in the literature of the 1930s and '40s and the slightly derogatory term *male menopause* from the 1960s onwards. More recently, it has become known as andropause or, better still, testosterone deficiency syndrome because it is being recognized at a wider age range and in association with other diseases such as diabetes.

It's as if nature has decided to rapidly reduce the possibility of reproduction after age fifty by causing the marker of fertility in women to cease, the periods, and in men by reducing erectile power generally, decreasing morning erections in particular. When life expectancy was around fifty, which it was in Europe and America in the 1920s and '30s (and still is in men in some countries such as Russia and parts of Africa), then the symptoms in men over that age were regarded as normal ageing.

Now that in many developed countries, healthy life expectancy, including a sexually active life for both sexes, has risen to over seventy and, in many, over eighty, the acceptable criteria of a good later life have changed.

Adding to this is the mounting evidence, particularly over the last ten years, that testosterone deficiency is associated with a host of serious physical diseases of later life, such as heart disease, obesity, diabetes, osteoporosis, and even Alzheimer's disease.

Faced with this evidence in an ageing population, you may think that doctors will be eager to encourage treatment for men complaining of the typical symptoms of testosterone deficiency syndrome. Not a bit of it. They seem to be leaning over backward not to make this particular diagnosis. Only 1 percent of the 20 percent of men over the age of fifty who have moderate to severe symptoms of the condition are diagnosed or treated.

Many endocrinologists rate the frequency of the condition as only 2 percent of the male population in the forty-to-eighty-year-old age range. If, as clinical experience and application of symptom questionnaires confirms, the figure is ten times greater, this is the most common hormonal disorder in men and yet the least frequently treated. Why does the orthodox medical establishment allow this to continue?

Firstly, they are entrenched in the dogma that to diagnose testosterone deficiency, there has to be a level of the hormone in the blood which is lower than the laboratory norm, together with symptoms.

This is regardless of the fact that all the studies using the standard questionnaire which covers these symptoms, the Ageing Male Symptom (AMS) questionnaire, show that there is little or no relationship between symptoms and testosterone levels. Therefore, you have to pick one or the other. Why insist on both when they are unrelated?

The usual reason given is that modern so-called scientific medicine prefers laboratory measurements rather than untidy things, like patient symptoms, regardless of the fact that it's the symptoms which make up the syndrome and cause the distress. Because the two don't correlate, clinicians say the symptom questionnaires are nonspecific. If you make the diagnosis from the symptomatic *syndrome* point of view, it's the lab tests which are nonspecific.

The lack of correlation between lab tests and the symptoms is due to several factors. The measurements made in the laboratory are largely invalid because the so-called normal ranges are variable between labs, countries, populations, and individuals. Lab values for testosterone can fall by 15–30 percent after food. It has recently been shown that Spanish men are archetypal 'high-T' guys so that like racing cars, they only feel and function well sexually on 'high-octane' hormonal fuel.

Lab results are also wrongly interpreted because they are log-normally distributed, but this technical point can drag a sufferer into the 'normal range' and deny him testosterone treatment. Those lab-centred physicians who base their dogma tent on the slippery slope of testosterone values are also faced with the uncomfortable fact that several studies have shown that *normal ranges* are decreasing decade by decade, so that on average, men have one-third less testosterone in the blood than their fathers at the same age.

Also, there is the key factor of testosterone resistance comparable to insulin resistance seen in adult-onset diabetics. This resistance to the production and action of testosterone is a new concept that has been overlooked by the medical profession in general because it makes it possible for a man to have normal or even high levels of testosterone but still be relatively deficient because of his needs at that time and have the corresponding symptoms accordingly.

Medical Insurance Companies and State Providers

Currently, most health insurance companies and state providers in the USA and UK cover neither HRT nor TRT and certainly don't want to do so. However severe the symptoms of the hormonal disturbances which endocrine lack can cause, they regard the resulting conditions as just due to ageing, even if they occur in midlife and can be reversed by economical hormonal treatments.

They think they have a strong financial incentive to

deny the existence of testosterone deficiency, the treatment costs of which in testosterone products alone, not counting the fees of the doctors administering it and the lab tests, is estimated at 2.2 billion USD annually, though it could and should be made much cheaper.

Certainly, some doctors and medical chains are more profit- than medical need-orientated, and it is difficult to regulate this, but limiting treatment to patients whose blood test show a low T is definitely not the way. In the process of trying to eliminate patients who do not need treatment, you will deny the large majority who do. History, symptoms, and full clinical assessment, I suggest, are the way forward. It works for HRT; why not TRT?

One troubling development is that several of the pharmaceutical companies marketing testosterone products in the USA use aggressive direct-to-consumer campaigns on television and other media, hyping the dangers of low T. This, as explained previously, is inaccurate in that because of resistance to its action, it is low T *activity* which is the problem. Also they have escalated the price of their products to make it an expensive treatment. This is unacceptable to both doctors and the insurance companies as testosterone itself is remarkably cheap to produce from its natural precursor, cholesterol. It's not produced from Peruvian bulls' testicles in the mating season, but from soy, which is cheap. With it having been available in pure crystalline form for over seventy years, there are little to no development costs, and so there is a very high profit margin.

For example, a month's supply in the UK of one of the most common forms of treatment, a gel preparation called Testogel, costs £30. In the USA, it is called AndroGel, comes in a pump dispenser rather than the more economical daily sachets, and costs 310 USD (£210) in the equivalent monthly dosage. This is sort of the markup designed to give testosterone treatment a bad name. It is an example of the practice by some pharmaceutical firms of 'price gouging'.

'Ageing Naturally' Arguments

There are many opponents of TRT who claim that it is just disease-mongering and choose to ignore the physical and mental benefits of the treatment, which are obvious to those who experience them, to their relatives, and to the doctors prescribing it. If the symptoms go away and stay away on treatment, recur when it is stopped even for a short period, and then go away again when it is resumed, this is not just a placebo effect.

There is a school of thought that adopts an almost moralistic ideology that we should learn to 'grow old gracefully' without medication to improve the quality of later life. This appears to ignore the reality that life expectancy from men has risen from forty-five in 1927 to fifty in 1950 and over eighty in 2000 but that most of this longevity is due to increased periods of frailty and dependency.

For many people, these are not enjoyable or productive years which they can live gracefully, but miserable and expensive ones for the individual and society alike. If you get angina and intermittent claudication pain in the legs, have diabetes and suffer from impaired mobility due to a fractured hip, and worst of all have to try to live with dementia, these are not desirable ways to grow old gracefully. Without medical intervention in the form of TRT for men and HRT for women, life can become an expensive burden. Ageing naturally sucks!

Also, particularly in America, there is the religious view that testosterone is all to do with sex, which is mainly for procreation, and is therefore immoral, unseemly, and unnecessary in those over the age of fifty. This ignores the fact that testosterone is not just a sex hormone but has physical functions in relation to body strength and vitality, energy, and enthusiasm.

Many of the same arguments, of course, apply to women, most of whom will like to spend their later life with active, happy, and healthy partners.

Myths of Testosterone Treatment

> *The great enemy of truth is very often not the lie – deliberate, contrived and dishonest – but the myth – persistent, persuasive and unrealistic. Too often we hold fast to the clichés of our forebears. We subject all facts to a prefabricated set of interpretations. We enjoy the comfort of opinion without the discomfort of thought.*
>
> John F. Kennedy,
> Commencement Address at Yale University, 11 June 1962

Nowhere in medicine has the power of myths had a greater influence in holding back progress in the introduction of a medical treatment than in the prominence given to the two great myths about testosterone treatment.

These myths are taught to fledgling medical students, who pass their exams and even get scholarships and awards for reciting them. They constitute fixed ideas in the minds of doctors and medical journalists whenever testosterone treatment is mentioned. Even when comprehensively disproved by the latest medical research, they are trotted out again and again. They resemble the regenerating life of vampires, who have to be nailed to the ground with the crucifix of a definitive rebuttal in a leading journal article. Even then, they are apt to rise again in the minds of older doctors and in articles by less-informed medical and lay journalists who haven't heard, or don't want to know, that their routinely regurgitated myth has been slain.

Myth Number 1: It May Cause Prostate Cancer

This was the big one that lasted over sixty years, since the idea was dreamt up by a famous American urologist called Charles Huggins. It was based on one patient of his with prostate cancer who appeared to get worse on testosterone replacement treatment (TRT) and temporarily better when treated with the female hormone estrogen, which suppressed release of the hormone.

This simplistic idea became enshrined in the anti-testosterone movement, and many prostate cancer victims were physically or chemically castrated to slow the growth of the tumor. This it did for a few months, but at the cost of bringing on the side effects of a testosterone-deficient state, with loss of libido, potency, and brain fog, which often severely reduced his quality of life.

This was seen in the sad closing chapter of a patient I saw at the Middlesex Hospital in London back in the 1960s. Shortly after a successful career as an eminent consultant physician, he developed prostate cancer, and as the urologist treating him worked at the hospital where the synthetic estrogen stilboestrol had been discovered by Sir Charles Dodds in the late 1930s, he was duly put on that drug.

Though it made him feel tired and forgetful, with florid symptoms of chemical testosterone deficiency, he lasted some months with only limited worsening of his prostate cancer, until he went to a family wedding and crashed head-on into another car, several of whose occupants were killed outright. He died depressed about the incident a few months later, a sad ending to an illustrious career.

Also, the idea seemed to ignore the fact that often, it is men with low testosterone levels who develop prostate cancer and that it only becomes common in men over the age of fifty, whose testosterone levels are falling naturally, who develop the condition. Also, intrepid patients using TRT for many years because of the general benefits they have experienced in losing their low-testosterone life and love-limiting symptoms obstinately refuse to develop prostate cancer above the rate experienced by the general population. It was a case of a beautiful theory slain by a few ugly facts. Undeterred, the medical establishment, whenever TRT was mentioned, would appear waving shrouds marked 'Whoa, beware, prostate cancer'.

It was not until a bold young American professor of urology at Harvard Medical School, Abe Morgentaler, developed a theory that there was a low threshold of testosterone above which there was no increased risk of cancer.

As he states in the summary of that article, 'studies have failed to show increased risk of PCa in men with higher serum T, and supraphysiologic T fails to increase prostate volume or prostate-specific antigen in healthy men. This apparent paradox is explained by the Saturation Model, which posits a finite capacity of androgen to stimulate PCa growth. Modern studies indicate no increased risk of PCa among men with serum T in the therapeutic range'.

'Fortunately,' Dr. Morgentaler concludes on his highly recommended website, Wellness Profile, and in his excellent new book, *Testosterone for Life*, 'all of these barriers are now relaxing, as it becomes clear how many body systems rely on healthy, normal T levels, and how normal T levels contribute to prevention of cardiovascular disease, diabetes, and the metabolic syndrome.'

He is even taking his ideas into his clinic, successfully treating some patients who are at high risk of prostate cancer or have had the condition and been treated for it with TRT. This is a complete reversal from the conventional wisdom that TRT is a complete taboo in prostate cancer cases to a situation where it can be judiciously alternated with androgen-deprivation treatment in advanced prostate cancer.

As he states in the summary of this article, 'this prohibition against T therapy has undergone recent re-examination with refinement of our understanding of the biology of androgens and PCa, and increased appreciation of the benefits of T therapy. A reassuringly low rate of negative outcomes has been reported with T therapy after radical prostatectomy (RP), radiation treatments, and in men on active surveillance. Although the number of these published reports are few and the total number of treated men is low, these experiences do provide a basis for consideration of T therapy in selected men with PCa. For clinicians considering offering this treatment, we recommend first selecting patients with low grade cancers and undetectable prostate-specific antigen following RP (Radical Prostatectomy).

'Further research is required to define the safety of T therapy in men with PCa. However, many patients symptomatic from T deficiency are willing to accept the potential risk of PCa progression or recurrence in return for the opportunity to live a fuller and happier life with T therapy'.

His detailed and scholarly attacks on the two main myths of testosterone treatment, that it causes prostate cancer and cardiovascular disease, have surely earned him the title of the 'mighty mythbuster'. The thanks of many patients worldwide and the doctors who treat them are due to him.

His experience coincides with that of consultant urologist Mark Feneley and myself in treating 2,500 patients with symptoms of androgen deficiency with TRT over twenty-five years at the Centre for Men's Health, with careful monitoring of the prostate. As reported in the leading *American Journal of Sexual Medicine* in 2012 with an article we dared to call 'Is Testosterone Treatment Good for the Prostate? Study of Safety During Long-Term Treatment' there is no increase in prostate cancer in men having TRT and no rise in the early warning marker, the prostate specific antigen (PSA).

Instead, many men show not only benefits in losing the symptoms of testosterone deficiency but also have improvement in lower urinary tract symptoms, such as frequency of passing water especially at night. This illustrates the point that TRT causes neither benign nor malignant prostate conditions but is good for the health of the entire urinary tract.

Myth Number 2: It May Cause Heart Disease

It seems that doctors enjoy a good myth. Perhaps it makes them seem more knowledgeable and stops them from having to practise a different form of medicine they know little or nothing about.

Just as the prostate cancer myth is in its death throes, a fresh myth is revived to take its place. Those that wish to block the use of TRT have switched their line of reasoning to the mistaken idea that it contributes to cardiovascular disease.

Nowhere is the pull of this second myth put forward more strongly than by advocates of consumer rights. The basic tenet of this movement is that the consumer, the patient in this case, has the unalienable right to the latest and best treatment without regard to its cost and without any possible side effects.

This view is usually put forward by people outside the medical profession, as those within it tend to have more reasonable expectations. Though believing that treatments and medication should be as safe as possible, they are aware from bitter experience that no treatment is perfectly safe and totally risk free. It is a constant risk–benefit analysis. Even aspirin used to treat your headache can very rarely cause you to bleed to death or have a hemorrhagic stroke which kills you.

In 2014, that bastion of orthodoxy, the *British Medical Journal*, to bolster its largely anti-testosterone stance, commissioned an article by the founder and director of a Washington-based organization called Public Citizen entitled 'Increased Heart Attacks in Men Using Testosterone: The UK Importantly Lags Far Behind the US in Prescribing Testosterone'. For the reasons to be discussed, the first part to this title is questionable, even though the second part is right, but not in the way the authors have intended. Because of restricted prescribing of testosterone in the UK, the US is way ahead in prescribing TRT.

Working initially with consumer rights activist Ralph Nader, Wolfe, aged seventy-five, and his organization Public Citizen, have worked to get twenty-five drugs off the market, pressured the Occupational Safety and

Health Administration to set tougher worker health standards, banned Red Dye No. 2, got warning labels about Reye's syndrome on aspirin bottles, and got silicone breast implants restricted, according to the release.

All very worthy causes and a much-needed watchdog over the FDA, especially since its funding was switched from public funding to pharmaceutical company sponsorship. Also, Donald Trump as President is now arguing for reduced FDA regulation to speed up the licensing of drugs and make them cheaper. However, this case is based on some dubious recent studies, and if this is the twenty-sixth drug they have taken up cause against, it may be one too far. Undeterred by twenty years of clinical studies showing benefits to the heart and circulation, opponents have based their recent attacks on rising sales figures for testosterone preparations in the US especially and the three flawed studies.

Back in 1945, when TRT was still gaining popularity, an American cardiologist reported that in ten patients, testosterone injections improved angina. Then there was a lull till, during the 1980s, a series of epidemiological articles suggested that low testosterone levels were associated with a greater risk of heart disease and that TRT lowered several risk factors, including blood pressure and cholesterol.

That TRT is beneficial to the heart and circulation was obvious to doctors who use this form of treatment with their patients suffering the classic symptoms of testosterone deficiency syndrome and related disorders. These include diabetes, obesity, metabolic syndrome, osteoporosis, and even Alzheimer's disease. A range of risk factors for heart disease, such as blood pressure, cholesterol, triglycerides, and abdominal obesity, are seen to decrease on the treatment, and especially in diabetics, there is a decrease in heart attack and mortality rates. Then, as seems inevitable with the cyclical nature of research and the varying hemlines of medical research, along comes TOM.

Following twenty years of clinical research showing TRT as being beneficial to the heart, especially in diabetics and in congestive heart failure, an American article alarmingly titled 'The TOM Study: Testosterone in Old Men' appeared in the prestigious *New England Journal of Medicine* in 2010.

This article, with an impressive list of no fewer than twenty-seven authors from Boston University Endocrinology Department, reports on a study conducted on 209 men sixty-five years or older, half over seventy-five, chosen on the basis of low testosterone levels. These men were not only elderly but also largely immobile, with difficulty even in climbing stairs and walking, but the usual symptoms of testosterone deficiency were not recorded, so we have no way of knowing whether they were really deficient or not, other than a very fallible random blood testosterone level.

The researchers then gave these frail, probably confused old men a complicated regime of three packets of testosterone gel or placebo to take, the dose regulated on the basis of blood levels after just two weeks rather than symptom relief, if any. This was likely to result in over-dosage in many of the subjects, especially if incorrectly applied. Also, there were more black people in the control group, and they were more prone to over-dosage. Baseline readings showed more men with high blood pressure and fat readings in the testosterone-treated group, both risk factors for heart disease.

The article also reported several highly unlikely findings: (1) no increased risk of adverse events up to a body mass index of 40 (morbidly obese), (2) diabetes and smoking halved the rate of adverse events, and (3) high baseline TT halved the risk, while high treatment TT doubled it. The authors themselves concluded, 'The small size of the trial and the unique population prevent broader inferences from being made about the safety of testosterone therapy.' These reservations unfortunately did not however appear in the press reports, and the journalists leapt to draw their own conclusions.

Many experts in testosterone treatment and cardiology agree that this was a thoroughly unsatisfactory study both in design and execution, best summarized as the subjects being too old, too frail, and on treatment likely to raise their testosterone too high.

Vigen Study

The second article frequently quoted is by Vigen et al. in *JAMA* in November 2013 entitled 'Association of Testosterone Therapy with Mortality, Myocardial Infarction, and Stroke in Men With Low Testosterone Levels'.

It economized in only having twelve authors but made up for it in being based on a vast retrospective study of 8,709 men from the Veterans Affairs system who were having coronary angiography between 2005 and 2011. The problem of such large groups is that there is very little data on each patient available for detailed assessment and that factors which are not clinically or biologically significant can be made statistically significant.

The approach of the authors is given in the summary, in that the stated importance of the article as given in the abstract was that it agreed with the concerns raised by the few previous adverse reports, not that it disagreed with most of the clinical studies over the previous twenty years.

To start with, it was unlikely that those having any sort of testosterone for even the briefest period had adequate or properly administered treatment. The testosterone started, on average, eighteen months after angiography and only lasted up to the cutoff point at three years, suggesting that half the time, patients in the treatment group were not on testosterone.

When they were, only 13 (1.1 percent) had what might be considered adequate and consistent treatment, testosterone gel. Of the 8,709 men with a total testosterone level lower than 300 ng/dL, 1,223 patients started testosterone therapy after a median of 531 days following coronary angiography. Of the 1,710 outcome events in this group of men at high risk of vascular disease, overall, 748 men died (8.5 percent), 443 had MIs (5.1 percent), and 519 (6.0 percent) had strokes. Of 7,486 patients not receiving testosterone therapy, 681 died (9.1 percent), 420 had MIs (5.6 percent), and 486 (6.5 percent) had strokes. Among 1,223 patients receiving testosterone therapy, 67 died (5.5 percent), 23 had MIs (1.9 percent), and 33 (2.7 percent) had strokes, simple statistics suggesting a clear benefit to the testosterone-treated group. These findings were reversed by the use of sophisticated statistics using stabilized inverse probability of weighting techniques and used to show the alleged dangers of TRT to the heart. This conforms to the old saying that if you torture statistics long enough, they will confess to anything.

The few adequately treated gel-treated patients were facing heroic odds when set against approximately 2.9 percent of men over the age of forty on TRT in the USA (nearly one and a half million) currently using the medication with sufficient benefit to wish to continue and without clinically obvious adverse side effects.

Expert clinicians in the field worldwide were left speechless and wrote letters of protest to the editor of *JAMA* and other journals and raged at conferences about the design of the study and the statistical analyses used. Where is the balance of evidence on which to issue such alarmist health warnings?

In summary, this study could be summarized as a study with too many patients and dubious statistical techniques used to reverse the initial findings.

The publicity over this article had an immediate adverse effect on the public image of TRT, which is continuing to this day. If you look up Google trends under interest in 'low testosterone' on the web you will see that before these articles in 2013 there was a peak of around 100 hits per day, which fell to 53 by the end of 2015. Many US physicians in the TRT field report a continuing halving of patients going on and staying on treatment. This echoes the lasting damage to the health of women on HRT caused by the now largely discredited Women's Health Initiative (WHI) study.

The myths surrounding these important and effective means of preventive medicine and treatment are having a deadly effect on their use.

PLOS ONE Study

Thirdly, a paper in a relatively seldom quoted and low-ranking, open-access journal, *PLOS ONE*, was published in January 2014 entitled 'Increased Risk of Non-Fatal Myocardial Infarction Following Testosterone Therapy Prescription in Men'.Following the other two studies and quoting them as reasons for this one, the mainly commercial statistician authors used insurance data on 55,593 men who filled a first prescription for any of several testosterone prescriptions. These included testosterone gel, micronized testosterone cypionate injections, and testosterone patches. Again, the numbers are so great that the clinically insignificant factors become statistically significant.

The main potential weakness of this trial is the control group of 167,279 men who took PDE5 inhibitors. This leads to confusion in the selection of a group who may have silent coronary disease and who are therefore completely unsuitable as a control group. Men who are known to have heart disease, especially those with angina, and on coronary vasodilator drugs are not supposed to take these drugs and would have been excluded by their physicians. These considerations alone should have invalidated the study and prevented it from being published.

Misled by studies such as the three above and their unjustified conclusions, the orthodox medical establishment and the general public are being unduly alarmed about the possibility of an association between testosterone treatment and circulatory disease.

Attempting to Trash the Case for Testosterone Treatment

This has long been a favorite technique for opponents of the treatment, especially when losing the scientific case. The most common approach is to use the following ten golden rules for trying to demolish the case for testosterone treatment:

1. *Start by invoking commercial greed and disease-mongering on the part of Big Pharma* as the cause of the large increase in testosterone prescriptions in North America. Produce alarming

statistics about US pharmaceutical sales of testosterone increasing from $324 million in 2002 to $2billion in 2012, and the number of testosterone prescriptions climbing from 100 million in 2002 to half a billion in 2012.

Impressive figures certainly, but how much of this increase is due to the effectiveness of direct-to-consumer product advertising (DTCPA) and how much to increased public awareness of the causes and symptoms of testosterone deficiency and increasing demand for the relief of these symptoms and associated conditions, such as osteoporosis and diabetes? This is combined with a reduced fear of prostate cancer among prescribers.

As has been pointed out by Prof. Abe Morgentaler in 2010 during the steepest increase in testosterone prescriptions, no testosterone product is within the top twenty most-advertised drugs. This suggests that Direct To Consumer Product Advertising (DTCPA) is only a partial explanation at best and a fat red herring at worst.

2. *Set your own standards for the diagnosis of 'late-onset hypogonadism' and ignore any evidence to the contrary.* Insist on the purely laboratory diagnosis of the condition based on low testosterone levels, regardless of the fallacies involved in doing so, and the lack of relationship of these with clinical symptoms and conditions or prognosis on treatment.
3. *Play up the myths* of dangers, such as prostate cancer and cardiovascular disease, even if these fears have been disproved. Ignoring thirty years' worth of evidence to the contrary, insist that there

is no convincing evidence that testosterone treatment of 'age-related hypogonadism' is safe.

4. *Associate the testosterone treatment* with other drugs of unproven benefit, such as growth hormone.
5. *Link TRT with the fallacious findings in relation to HRT arising from the Women's Health Initiative (WHI) study* even if the findings of that mainly one product study has largely been disproved.
6. *Associate testosterone deficiency purely with ageing* and maintain that treating it is therefore unjustified and meddling with nature. While choosing your own terms carefully, remember at all times that by definition, 'age-related hypogonadism' is a rare condition diagnosed on the basis of an assumed normal distribution of testosterone at different ages of 0.5 percent rather than the 40 percent of the over forty-fives suggested by some authors who take more account of symptoms.
7. *March under the banner of science-based medicine* even if it is in fact opinion based and this basis crumbles under closer scrutiny.
8. *Dismiss all opponents of your views* as disease-mongering permissive prescribers using lax, distorted clinical judgement. The terms *quackery* and *hucksterism* are useful here. In other words, deride all those practising outside the true faith of so-called modern scientific medicine however fallible and incomplete that science may be. Whatever the results they get and however satisfied their patients are, they are heretics rather than 'disease-mongering'. Refusing to accept that many men after the age of fifty, particularly those with symptoms, could be suffering from reduced testosterone

activity, and might benefit from treatment, is 'disease denial' and bad medical practice.

9. *Join with others* who have similar views to your own and form a chorus of opposition.
10. *Air your views loudly* and repetitively at conferences and in journal articles, obeying Lewis Carroll's dictum in the hunting of the Snark, 'What I tell you three times is true' however apparently nonsensical it proves when carefully analyzed.

To show how worthless these ten golden rules are, I suggest you consider the following logic.

Testosterone levels are largely invalid as measures of testosterone deficiency because of the following:

1. *Preanalytical factors* (The exact sampling conditions in relation to circadian and seasonal variations, diet, alcohol, physical activity, and posture)
2. *Physiological and medical factors* (Androgen levels vary according to the patient's biological age, his physical and mental health, stress, sexual activity, and smoking habits.)
3. *Analytical variables* (Sample preservation and storage are often unknown, different androgen assays have widely different accuracy and precision and are subject to large interlaboratory variation exhortations to use GCMS, and take multiple samples that are expensive and often impractical in routine clinical practice.)
4. *Interpretation of results* (Laboratory reference ranges vary widely, largely independent of methodology, and fail to take into account the log-normal distribution of androgen values, all causing errors in clinical diagnosis and treatment.)

5. *Internal androgen resistance* (Impaired androgen synthesis or regulation, increased androgen binding, reduced tissue responsiveness, decreased androgen receptor activity, impaired transcription and translation)

There is no relationship between testosterone levels and symptoms, associated conditions, and the response to testosterone treatment. This is hardly surprising in view of the first two factors but is totally ignored by those bent on denying testosterone treatment to patients.

Consequences of Testosterone Resistance

The reality of testosterone resistance is that it is a game changer; it changes the thinking about the causes, diagnosis, and treatment of testosterone deficiency.

What Testosterone Resistance Means in Terms of Diagnosis

> *There are two ways to be fooled. One is to believe what isn't true; the other is to refuse to believe what is true.*
>
> Søren Kierkegaard, Danish Philosopher, 1813–1855

Most of the opponents of testosterone treatment cleverly manage to make both errors at the same time.

This new idea of testosterone resistance means going back to the drawing board for both the diagnosis and treatment of testosterone deficiency.

Once you have accepted the principle, the evidence for its existence and importance falls into place.

Firstly, the idea that blood tests are the gold standard for deciding whether a man is deficient falls by the wayside. When you examine the sampling problems, the laboratory measurement problems, and the interpretation problems, you realize that far from being the measure of the condition, it is fool's gold. It is not low T, as the adverts say, but low T activity, a very different thing.

So out go all the ideas of screening campaigns for finding low testosterone levels in the community in favor of making men aware of the symptoms of testosterone deficiency and helping them recognize the key features. They should seek help if and when they need it or develop a related condition such as diabetes. You won't suggest screening for the menopause in women, will you?

By all means, measure the testosterone levels once the diagnosis has been established on a symptomatic basis, preferably using Prof. Lothar Heineman's excellent Ageing Male Symptoms (AMS) questionnaire. This is available free in twenty languages, has been fully validated, and is also available online (www.andropause.org.uk). This simple but effective diagnostic tool is also given in full, together with the scoring system, at the end of this book. The seventeen questions are each rated 1–5, and a total score of over 37 makes the diagnosis of testosterone deficiency moderately likely, and over 50 highly probable.

When the AMS questionnaire was completed in a web survey by over 10,000 men, mainly from the UK and USA, 80 percent who responded had moderate or severe scores, likely to benefit from TRT. The average age of these men was fifty-two, many cases in their forties, an age when the diagnosis of so-miscalled 'late-onset hypogonadism' is not generally considered. Other possible contributory factors to the high testosterone deficiency scores reported were obesity (29 percent), alcohol (17.3 percent), testicular problems such as mumps orchitis

(11.4 percent), prostate problems (5.6 percent), urinary infection (5.2 percent), and diabetes (5.7 percent).

It was concluded that in this self-selected large international sample of men, there was a very high prevalence of scores which would warrant a therapeutic trial of testosterone treatment. The study suggested that there are large numbers of men in the community whose testosterone deficiency was neither being diagnosed nor treated.

The lack of relationship between blood testosterone levels and the symptoms has been clearly shown in the UK Androgen Study of men presenting for TRT with symptoms of deficiency over the last twenty-five years to establish the symptom response when testosterone treatment was initiated on the basis of clinical features and symptoms of androgen deficiency and the resulting endocrine, biochemical, and physiological responses.

Of 2,693 patients attending the three Men's Health Centres (The UK Androgen Study (UKAS)), 2,247 were treated. Treatments included pellet implants, oral testosterone undecanoate (Testocaps), mesterolone (Proviron), testosterone gel (Testogel), testosterone scrotal cream (Andromen), and scrotal gel (Tostran).

There was no correlation between initial testosterone level, initial symptom score, or the success of treatment as defined by adequate resolution of symptoms. Despite the diverse endocrine patterns produced, the testosterone preparations appear equally safe over prolonged periods, with either no change or improvement of cardiovascular risk factors, especially in lowering cholesterol and diastolic blood pressure.

However, the initial findings clearly showed that there was no significant increase in total symptom scores over the full range of total and free testosterone.

Also, the initial level of testosterone was no use in assessing whether the patient would respond to treatment or not. Those who started on treatment with symptoms and a high total testosterone responded just as well as those that might have been diagnosed on the basis of their low total testosterone. In other words, total testosterone is of no use in diagnosis or prognosis.

Other researchers have confirmed the way that testosterone levels are not related to symptoms, but still they are used as the basis of the diagnosis of testosterone deficiency. Take for example these quotations from the summaries of their articles:

1. 'There was no correlation between AMS (total and subscales) and testosterone levels.'
2. 'None of the three AMS domain scale scores significantly correlated with testosterone, free testosterone or bioavailable testosterone. Significant correlations were observed between results for the AMS scores and those for other health questionnaires, but none of the subscores for the latter questionnaires correlated with androgen serum levels.'
3. 'None of the three AMS domain scale scores and total scores significantly correlated with serum levels of TT, FT, E2, LH, FSH, DHEA-S, or GH.'
4. 'The lack of correlation between the clinical picture and the most commonly used biochemical confirmatory tests (TT, SHBG, LH), again, clearly points to the paramount importance of the clinical evaluation. An emphasis and reliance on serum T alone hinders the clinician's ability to manage testosterone deficiency syndromes (TDS).'

5. 'A problem with the diagnosis of LOH (Late Onset Hypogonadism) is that often the symptoms (in 20–40% of unselected men) and low circulating T (in 20% of men >70 years of age) do not coincide in the same individual.' By combining these criteria 'only 2% of 40- to 80-year-old men have LOH.' Nice one, this, though the logic is unclear. Why, if the two diagnostic tests for a condition don't agree, then insist on using both of them together?
6. 'The search for a discrete threshold may be futile given emerging evidence. Recent studies suggest that testosterone threshold varies by symptoms and among individuals. In addition, thresholds may vary between young and old men. Therefore, initiation of treatment should rely more on symptoms and less on a discrete numerical threshold.'

Diagnosing according mainly to blood testosterone levels as measured before treatment is also guaranteed to miss a large proportion of cases of testosterone deficiency. This was shown by looking at the testosterone levels in over 2,000 patients in my practice who presented with symptoms and had marked relief of these symptoms when treated with testosterone.

Only 2% of these patients had testosterones below the level they would need to get treatment under the Pharmaceutical Benefit Scheme in Australia (6 nmol/l). A generous 17% would get treated in the UK under the NHS and in most European countries at 12nmol/l. Not until the level of about 27 nmol/L is reached would all symptomatic cases included as being eligible for treatment.

Looked at another way, what clinician would decide

his clinical practice on the basis of a test which appears to have a false-negative rate of over 80 percent?

Treating Testosterone Deficiency

The idea of testosterone resistance profoundly alters the approach to both diagnosis and treatment. In treating a man with symptoms of testosterone deficiency or a related condition such as diabetes, you not only have to raise the testosterone level but also consider ways of reducing resistance to its action. As in diabetes, you are treating either an absolute or relative deficiency of a hormone.

Testing for Testosterone Resistance

Firstly, though you don't need to do it routinely, you can test for testosterone resistance. You can suspect it in most cases, certainly below the age of fifty, by the high level of testosterone in the presence of clear symptoms. Where this is not the case, you can confirm the resistance by a therapeutic trial of an injection of a long-acting preparation, such as testosterone undecanoate (Nebido in the UK and Europe (1 g), Reandron in Australia (1 g), or Aveed in the USA (0.75 g)).

The 1 g injections are designed to last up to three months, where there is low resistance as in young men with primary testicular failure, nondescent, or orchidectomy for testicular cancer. Too often, urological surgeons removing one testis pat their young patients on the back and say, 'You still have the other testis. You'll be fine.' But within two or three years, they develop symptoms of testosterone deficiency, which are frequently not recognized or are ignored rather than relieved by TRT as part of the routine follow-up.

However, the typical patient in their fifties notice that their symptoms improve for a shorter time after the 1 g injection, say, six weeks, so that what could be called the testosterone resistance index (TRI) is 12/6, i.e. 2, rather than 12/12, i.e. 1. This is where the resistance is often due to multiple causes such as age, stress, alcohol, medications, or diabetes.

This test is simple to carry out and, if positive, can be followed by whatever treatment the clinician finds most effective. It can be compared to the glucose tolerance test for diabetics.

Testosterone Replacement Therapy (TRT)

The choice of testosterone treatment is much wider than it was twenty-five years ago, as considered in my article on 'The Evolution of Testosterone Treatment', with more options in the UK and Australia than in the USA.

Each of the seven different forms of testosterone treatment used over the previous twenty-five years can prove clinically effective when the patients are selected on the basis of the diagnostic symptoms, and to paraphrase the saying from George Orwell's *Animal Farm*, all treatments are equal, but some are more equal than others. It depends largely on the degree of resistance, costs of maintaining the treatment, and the patient's and clinician's preferences.

Treatments include pellet implants, oral testosterone undecanoate (Testocaps), mesterolone (Proviron), testosterone gel (Testogel), testosterone undecanoate injections (Nebido), testosterone scrotal cream (Andromen), and scrotal gel (Tostran). With the exception of mesterolone, which only has a weak therapeutic action, all treatments appear effective and safe, but the being so much better absorbed, the scrotal preparations have considerable price advantages.

Reducing the Resistance to Testosterone

Raising testosterone levels to overcome the resistance has been the mainstay of treatment since testosterone became available over seventy years ago. However, this does not overcome the root cause, may reduce the body's natural testosterone production, and needs to be maintained lifelong. Many of the measures needed to do so come under the heading of lifestyle modification, seldom an easy thing to achieve.

However, TRT creates a window of opportunity by boosting willpower and 'won't power', that he will reduce his intake of sugar and starches and won't snack, that he will take more exercise and become less of a couch potato. Results can be slow, but over a one year, studies have shown that patients can develop improved musculature and lose weight.

Weight Reduction

It's the old 'calories in, calories out' equation. Reducing and decreasing the portion and size and switching away from sugar and carbohydrate toward protein and vegetable oils are the bases. The Atkins diet series of books are very good for helping this process and are thoroughly recommended. A dietary pact with your partner can be very helpful here.

Alcohol is a key source of calories and can sap morale as well as generate stress. Beer also contains xenoestrogens and can cause weight gain.

Exercise should be gentle and progressive, vigorous but not violent, and dynamic rather than static. Walking for ten, fifteen, twenty minutes per day is a good start and can reduce stress levels, especially if undertaken with a dog. Cycling and rowing on a rowing machine are also suitable, noncompetitive forms of exercise for those over fifty.

Swimming is a particularly good form of exercise. You can be said to get double-bubble benefit with swimming. It is the right type of whole-body exercise, and you are burning off extra calories even in comfortably warm water.

A personal exercise trainer can be a good investment if you can afford it.

Stress Reduction

As well as directly reducing testosterone production, stress creates testosterone resistance by causing the release of the stress hormones epinephrine (adrenaline), norepinephrine (noradrenaline), cortisol, and a pituitary gland hormone called prolactin.

Rather than relying on drugs to reduce stress, stress-reduction methods should be employed within the limits of your lifestyle – not becoming a stress-avoiding vegetable but becoming aware of the performance-arousal curve.

This views stress as a force like electricity in your life. A certain amount is necessary to stimulate you and help you perform at your optimal level. It's when you go into overload that it can cause you to blow a fuse and burn out. You need to know and accept whether you are a thirty-amp-cooker-fuse type of person or a possibly more creative three-amp-lighting-fuse sort of person (figure 1).

Adequate sleep, which is the time when most testosterone is secreted, is essential to help you resist stress. This needs to be naturally obtained and not with the help of sleeping pills. This requires a regime of sleep-hygiene, involving a regular bedtime, no caffeinated drinks after 6:00 p.m., only one or two alcoholic drinks generally per evening, and switching off your exposure to computers and violent, worrying TV programs and films late at night. Sorry, but your brain needs to wind its activity down an hour or so before you go to sleep.

The many-millennia-old solution to stress through meditation is an ideal antidote to stress and is becoming very popular both in the UK and US. This involves sitting in a quiet place and simply turning one's attention within. You don't have to change your religion as many forms are nonsectarian. Christian prayer, Buddhist and Hindu mantra meditations, and even breath-watching, mindful meditation can all prove very relaxing and improve your experience of life. Meditation, not medication, should be your aim.

My personal choice is Siddha Meditation (perfect meditation), an ancient nonsectarian form which is taught free of charge at over 300 centres worldwide.

What is the way ahead in in increasing the use of testosterone treatment? Firstly, we stick with our medical colleagues who are quietly getting on with high-quality research showing the benefits of TRT in a wide range of conditions, including diabetes, obesity, metabolic syndrome, and even Alzheimer' s disease.

Secondly, and probably more importantly, given the testosterone resistance of the medical establishment and providing authorities and their entrenched opposition to TRT, we must enlist the help of what I call the patient's voice. This is the vast number of men experiencing the typical symptoms of testosterone deficiency as measured by the AMS questionnaire and comparing it with the experience of the relatively few men who have managed to get treatment for these symptoms.

This was the experience of over 10,000 men, mainly from the UK (70 percent) and USA (10 percent), who filled in the AMS questionnaire online on three different UK-based websites in 2011. Among them, 80 percent had moderate or severe scores suggesting that they would be likely to benefit from TRT. The average age of these men was fifty-two, with many cases in their forties, an age when the diagnosis of late-onset hypogonadism was not generally considered. Other possible contributory factors to the high testosterone deficiency scores reported were obesity (29 percent), alcohol (17.3 percent), testicular problems such as mumps orchitis (11.4 percent), prostate problems (5.6 percent), urinary infection (5.2 percent), and diabetes (5.7 percent).

From this large-scale study it was concluded that in this self-selected international sample of men, there was a very high prevalence of scores which would warrant a therapeutic trial of testosterone treatment. The study suggests that there are large numbers of men in the community whose testosterone deficiency is neither being diagnosed nor treated. The large number of men responding to the questionnaire and giving high scores has not abated since that study was carried out, and a follow-up is planned to see what has happened to these very largely untreated men and increase awareness of their unsolved problem.

Thirdly, given the vast number of untreated men round the world likely to be suffering the symptoms and side effects of testosterone deficiency, we have to acknowledge that it doesn't take a high powered consultant andrologist, endocrinologist or urologist to diagnose and treat the condition. A well trained general practitioner willing to follow the simple guidelines for diagnosing testosterone deficiency and monitoring the patient's progress can easily use the treatment in the majority of cases. In the process they can enjoy the satisfaction of often giving the man a new lease of healthy life.

Let's just encourage those willing to look at the wide-ranging but usually totally ignored evidence that

TRT can help in the prevention and treatment of the following conditions:

1. Symptoms of testosterone deficiency
2. Erectile dysfunction
3. Diabetes and its complications
4. Cardiovascular disease and preventing heart failure
5. Peripheral vascular disease and preventing gangrene
6. Some stages of prostate cancer
7. AIDS (HIV infections)
8. Depression
9. Early Alzheimer's disease
10. Parkinson's disease
11. Multiple sclerosis
12. Trauma to the head and spinal cord
13. Osteoporosis
14. Frailty of ageing
15. Prolongation of life

Of course, it's not a panacea, but given the above it would seem to be as good a candidate as any current drug can claim to be. Sometimes, this term is taken to mean a cure for a large, multifaceted problem, which, in the case of metabolic syndrome, with its combination of diabetes, lipid disturbances, and hypertension, it certainly seems to come close to.

Of course, skeptics will find studies that appear to deny its benefit in these conditions, but I will suggest that the weight of evidence is strongly in its favour. You are invited to look up reference libraries such as PubMed, and decide for yourself where the balance of evidence lies in any or all these conditions that interest you.

To finish on a hopeful note in this turbulent tale of the

fight for testosterone treatment, at a meeting in October 2015 of the International Society for the Study of the Ageing Male (ISSAM), there was a consensus conference on testosterone deficiency and its treatment, chaired by Prof. Abe Morgentaler, a urologist from Boston, and Prof. Michael Zitzman, an endocrinologist from München in Germany. The eighteen strong groups of international experts debated and agreed on the following resolutions:

1. Testosterone deficiency (TD) is a well-established, significant medical condition that negatively affects male sexuality, reproduction, and quality of life.
2. Symptoms and signs of TD occur as a result of low levels of testosterone and may benefit from treatment regardless if there is an underlying etiology.
3. TD is a global public health concern.
4. Testosterone therapy for men with TD is effective, rational, and evidence-based.
5. There is no T concentration that reliably distinguishes those who will respond to treatment from those who will not.
6. There is no scientific basis for recommendations against the use of T therapy in men over sixty-five years.
7. The evidence does not support increased risks of cardiovascular events with T therapy.
8. The evidence does not support increased risk of prostate cancer with T therapy.
9. Current evidence supports a major research initiative to explore possible benefits of T therapy for cardiometabolic disease.

The consensus agreement on these nine key points by these world experts, none of whom were influenced by pharmaceutical company sponsorship, was put forward to a press conference the same afternoon and gave great encouragement for the over 300 conference delegates who were coming to hear the latest news on TRT, its safety, and its effectiveness.

It seems only by the mobilization of public opinion in support of testosterone treatment, and the gradual overcoming of establishment resistance to the treatment by the already massive accumulation of favorable clinical evidence, that TRT will come to be seen as great an advance in preventive and therapeutic medicine for the twenty-first century as HRT was for women in the twentieth century.

This is best seen as the intended prolongation of healthy life so that men can live their life in square wave form, like alkaline batteries going full charge to the end (see Figure 1).

In this chapter we will see how at present, the established 'magical laws' of medicine are winning hands down over the natural desire of the doctor to do some good in the world.

Mukherjee puts forward three very practical new laws which seem to apply to the theme of this book. We will take each in turn.

Law 1: A Strong Intuition Is Much More Powerful than a Weak Test

Certainly, in the diagnosis of testosterone deficiency, the doctor's overall assessment, combined with his detailed, standardized symptom questionnaire, is far better than the currently favored total testosterone measured in the blood, or any other lab test come to that.

The total testosterone well fits the definition of a weak test as it is inaccurate, is misleading, misses up to 90 percent of cases that can benefit from treatment, and denies treatment to millions of men worldwide with the identikit symptoms of testosterone deficiency.

Law 2: 'Normals' Teach Us Rules, Outliers Teach Us Laws

Based on lab tests, usually total testosterone, most doctors try and achieve a Procrustean fit for the patient within the so-miscalled normal range of lab values. Outliers on this scale teach us the law that you can have rampant and health-threatening symptoms of testosterone deficiency yet have high levels of testosterone.

Like the high levels of insulin in some diabetic patients, a high level of testosterone well up or even above the so-called normal range can coexist with severe symptoms of deficiency which are rapidly cured by giving TRT, teaching us the law of testosterone resistance.

Also, when a young man in his thirties with advanced disease of the arteries of both legs, which has failed to respond to extensive surgery and where amputation appears the only answer, responds dramatically to TRT, ignore him. He is an outlier. When he is skiing and teaching tai chi on both legs twenty-five years later as one patient of mine was, still on high-dose TRT, he can safely be ignored as an outlier and, worse still, an embarrassment to his surgeons, who have made the diagnosis of hopeless progressive arterial disease and advised amputation.

Law 3: For Every Perfect Medical Experiment There Is a Perfect Human Bias

This certainly applies to research into testosterone treatment, where for every one of the thousands of encouraging trials showing the positive effects of TRT in relief of symptoms, coronary heart disease, osteoporosis, frailty, and debility, you can find a few negative ones. These are usually based on opinion rather than fact, which will criticize, deny, or oppose it. We have looked at the many of the sources of this bias against TRT in this book.

As a result of the application and distortion of the 'magical laws' conjured up by modern super-scientific medicine, I frankly think we are going in reverse as far as the availability of testosterone treatment is concerned both in the UK and in the US and, worst of all, in Australia.

This is similar to the turning of the tide of medical and, consequently, public opinion against HRT by two highly publicized studies which were published early this century and, looking back, appeared designed to create a climate of fear as described in the first chapter, the first being the Women's Health Initiative in the USA and the second the Million Women study in the UK.

The Million Women Study appeared in 2003 in that bastion of orthodoxy, *The Lancet*. Not only did the study make no allowance for women changing from their original form of HRT, but a review in 2011 also reported that the findings did not satisfy the criteria of time order, information bias, cofounding, statistical stability and strength of association, duration response, internal consistency, external consistency, or biological plausibility. The criticism seemed damning, but the damage to HRT had been done.

Typical of this hardening of the forces resistant to the

use of testosterone for the treatment of what they will insist terming *age-related hypogonadism* is the latest pronouncement of the Federal Drug Administration (FDA) in the *New England Journal of Medicine*. After reiterating the causes of relatively rare classic hypogonadism with obvious testicular malfunction, the authors make the interesting statement that the FDA only require that testosterone products 'reliably bring low serum concentrations into the normal range for healthy young men'.

This makes two fundamental erroneous assumptions within the first paragraph of the article. Firstly is that the condition can be defined in terms of testosterone levels at any age regardless of testosterone resistance. Secondly, that the aim of treatment is to bring serum concentrations to within the normal range for young men, whatever that may be. The aim of treatment for most practising clinicians is not to achieve any particular arbitrary level of testosterone but to alleviate the patient's symptoms or associated conditions.

What they go on to describe is the controversial condition that the FDA calls age-related or late-onset hypogonadism, even if it occurs in men in their forties, which may cause men over that age, expecting to live twice as long, to object. Then comes the traditional charge that in these cases, it is unclear (for which read we don't believe) 'whether co-existing nonspecific signs and symptoms, such as decreases in energy and muscle mass, are a consequence of the age-related decline in endogenous testosterone or whether they are a result of other factors, such as coexisting conditions, concomitant medications, or perhaps aging itself'.

For the many reasons already given, it is not the highly characteristic symptoms, which are nonspecific, but the unrelated and highly fallible blood testosterone levels, which, except in extreme cases, are nonspecific.

Following the traditional plea that not enough is known about the risks of TRT and a brief review of the conflicting studies on whether or not there may be increased risk of cardiovascular disease, big advisory organizations in September 2014 convened an advisory committee – which they usually do when they want to delay making a decision – saying that 'the available evidence supports an indication for testosterone therapy only in men with classic hypogonadism and that drug labels should state that the efficacy and safety of testosterone products have not been established for age-related hypogonadism. In addition, because there is no evidence of laboratory testing before the initial testosterone prescription for some men, committee members recommended adding a statement to drug labels about the need to confirm low serum testosterone concentrations before initiating treatment'.

Effectively, the FDA has taken it upon themselves to define *testosterone deficiency* in terms of low testosterone and pulls the rug from under any physician who dares to disagree. They then strike a dangerous blow to the future of TRT by requiring manufacturers of testosterone products to band together to conduct a long-term controlled clinical trial to 'better determine the effects of testosterone therapy on cardiovascular outcomes among users'.

This, as the FDA probably well know, is a complete nonstarter for several reasons. Firstly, why should highly competitive pharmaceutical rivals making a wide variety of testosterone preparations pour millions of dollars into any one product and limit sales for up to ten years to come up with results which are unlikely to be more conclusive than the results already found in expensive controlled trials before marketing? It sounds like what will be described in politics as a filibuster, a meaningless exercise just to induce delay while patients badly needing treatment go without.

Also, the routine academic cry at the end of every publication of 'more research before we can routinely recommend this treatment' means that in fact, we want to sit on the fence and do nothing except award ourselves and our coworkers big long-term research grants and continue to go to conferences in nice places indefinitely.

By contrast with this academic procrastination, let me give you an example of what can currently be achieved with testosterone treatment. With a couple of knowledgeable academic colleagues, I published a paper in a highly rated journal in the field after a year of writing and review by three referees who caused considerable revision of the paper. It was a review of clinical experience over twenty-five years using seven different forms of testosterone treatment at the three Centres for Men's Health in London, Manchester, and Edinburgh. It was probably the biggest and longest such study in the world involving over 2,000 men, giving in total over 4,500 man-years of experience.

It clearly showed several original findings. It showed the diverse hormonal changes associated with each treatment, yet there was sustained relief of the characteristic symptoms with each of them. The treatment was safe and in fact beneficial to the prostate, as had been shown in a previous analysis of the findings, with no increase in either benign or malignant changes in the prostate as reported in a previous paper. Neither were there any adverse changes in cardiovascular risk factors on the treatments. In fact, there were some beneficial changes in terms of significant reductions in cholesterol and blood pressure. The article also showed how the cost of treatment could be reduced to less than that of antidepressants, a most cheering and encouraging finding.

Intriguingly, it again showed that there was no relationship between testosterone levels before starting treatment and either symptoms of testosterone deficiency or the likelihood of a good response to treatment. It also showed that using pretreatment testosterone levels as cutoff points to decide which symptomatic cases should have the benefits of treatment resulted in over 90 percent of cases missing out.

You might have thought that the medical establishment might have welcomed this clarification of to whom and how to give testosterone treatment as based on extensive experience of testosterone treatment, but not a bit of it. Immediately, the article, when reported in the popular press, was greeted by those who might be described as the usual suspects with the following damning criticisms:

1. Firstly, they made a concerted effort to rubbish the study by describing it as being 'below the normal standards of science' since it was not a double blind controlled trial. However, this response raised the question of whether it was ethical to conduct such a trial of a group of medications which you knew could immediately transform the lives of people suffering the clear symptoms of a life-wrecking disease which can easily, rapidly, and safely be reversed, as many short-term, more academically correct studies had shown over the last seventy years since testosterone first became available.

   Also, if the referees of a specialist journal in the field, after careful review, had decided it should be published, who were the critics to say it should not be and ignore twenty-five years of carefully documented clinical evidence?

2. The critics then went on to say that the authors were obviously unaware of the expert guidelines saying that testosterone treatment should only be prescribed according to the threshold values of testosterone that had been set in stone by international organizations setting the condition's rules for treatment.

   My answer to that would be that testosterone values had been shown to be subject to up to 100 percent variation according to sampling and laboratory factors, as well as interpretation, and were totally unreliable as a basis for diagnosing testosterone deficiency. If they were, I would not be arguing in favor of using clinical history and symptoms as basis for the diagnosis of testosterone deficiency. So over the years, I had spent many hours studying and comparing various guidelines and, on the subject of criteria for the diagnosis of testosterone deficiency, could place little or no faith in cutoff levels of testosterone.

   Then of course, there are the factors in internal resistance to the action of any given level of testosterone, which I have described previously.

   I know that modern, evidence-based scientific medicine much prefers laboratory values to questionnaires as for the diagnosis of disease, but there is loads of scientific evidence that this is not the situation in the diagnosis of testosterone deficiency. Unfortunately, there is no lab test that gives a reliable diagnosis of testosterone deficiency any more than there is a test for depression. Depressing, but that's the way it is.

3. Critics also say that the study was 'misleading and potentially dangerous'. Well, it is only misleading if you believe that the level of testosterone in the blood is the main arbiter of treatment and wish to argue against the principle of testosterone resistance and the variability of symptoms of symptoms in relation to the level of testosterone, which was carefully explained in the article and carefully evidenced. It is curious that the very academics who say the treatment is dangerous are the ones who, twenty years ago, were proving its safety as a male contraceptive in doses two to three times higher than usually used for routine TRT.

   The same people will go on to give as an example of the dangers a rise in red blood cell numbers, called polycythemia, which occurred in one overdosed case treated with short-acting testosterone injections and not properly monitored. These injections are no longer used by any reputable expert in the field, precisely because they give a rollercoaster ride in symptoms rather than the smooth improvement that the daily treatments or long-lasting injections usually give. This however is more of a risk than other factors and should be carefully monitored throughout on any course of TRT.

4. Next up, the critics ignore the fact that the authors have moved on from calling the typical symptom complex the male menopause to the preferable and less-ageist term testosterone deficiency syndrome. They refer back to the thirty-year-old argument

that unlike the abrupt drop in estrogens occurring about the age of fifty at the menopause in women, there is only a 0.4 percent drop in testosterone in the age of thirty onwards. Mind you, that is an admitted 12 percent in what are average figures by age sixty, when, because of increasing testosterone resistance, this can make a critical difference to its action.

Also, there is the interesting fact that two studies, one in America and one in Finland, show that overall testosterone levels in the male population are falling quite rapidly and alarmingly to the point where young men have the same levels as that of their twenty- to thirty-years-older fathers. This may be due to increasing rates of obesity, scrotal warming in tighter trousers, environmental estrogens, and even pesticides. Whatever the causes, which may be multiple, both testosterone levels and sperm counts are falling in many countries till we have nearly reached a tipping point, where population numbers start to decrease.

Because the 0.4 percent is only an average figure and common factors in a man's life such as stress, alcohol, and increasing abdominal obesity, combined with decreasing fitness, can cause this drop to be greater and more rapid in the (at least) 20 percent of men over the age of fifty who develop the typical symptoms, slow decline in testosterone levels is a faulty argument even if routinely trotted out.

5. Then comes the argument that the main reason some older men have low testosterone levels is not the so-called manopause but underlying problems

such as obesity and age-related illnesses such as type 2 diabetes and heart failure. Heavy drinking, stress, depression, and medication – including certain painkillers – can also lower T levels. 'We men are hardwired to shut down testosterone levels when we are ill,' opponents explain. 'In these cases, it is the underlying problem which needs treatment, not the low testosterone levels.'

This is the chicken-and-egg argument. Is it the illness causing the low testosterone or the low testosterone causing the illness? Why not give testosterone and find out?

Well, except for the fact we have shown that it is not the level of testosterone which is the decisive factor in whether symptoms of testosterone deficiency develop and the illnesses quoted both lower testosterone levels and increase resistance to its action, saying that he won't need the help of testosterone treatment to overcome them seems faintly punitive and ridiculous.

6. Then comes the claim that the increasing use of testosterone treatment, as in America, where sales have increase by a factor of tenfold in the last ten years, must be due to disease-mongering rather than legitimate prescribing by doctors increasingly aware of true testosterone deficiency symptoms and the relief that TRT can provide. This is again based on making the diagnosis by the level of testosterone in the blood rather than on symptoms and their relief. Rigid application of a totally irrelevant test can be called disease denial, blatantly refusing to recognize testosterone deficiency symptoms as a means of denying TRT to the millions of men needing it.

Twenty years ago, at a meeting on men's health, when asking one such denier why GPs were failing to treat these manifest symptoms, he asserted that GPs were the gatekeepers of the NHS and were charged with keeping the hordes of men who might demand treatment away from such a dangerous and, in his opinion, unnecessary therapeutic trial. I then replied that I thought in this case the GPs were slamming the gate in the faces of the men needing treatment. Not surprisingly, it didn't go down well.

7. Then they subtly play the outdated 'danger of prostate cancer' card, often with an advertisement for a prostate cancer charity. They suggest that TRT can increase PSA, which it may do in the early stages of treatment in severely testosterone-deficient men, while it remains in the normal range for many years of treatment afterward. Also, which they don't mention, it definitely does not increase prostate cancer risks, as a previous UKAS study, along with many others, has shown.
8. Next, they routinely quote the faulty studies on TRT causing heart disease, which we have already demolished, but hey ho, on we go! Why muzzle the attack dogs?
9. Finally, they exaggerate the claims that even the most enthusiastic proponents of TRT may, but actually don't, make to say 'TRT is definitely not a cure-all'. 'What man of my age wouldn't want to put on muscle?' he asks. 'Who wouldn't want to be reborn?' It's the old panacea trick and quite unworthy of serious scientific debate.

Chapter 3 – HRT for Women

The average age of onset of the symptoms of menopause is near enough 50. This is the time to consult the health professional of your choice – don't leave it! Symptoms usually start a few months or years before periods stop, known as the perimenopause, and can persist for some time afterwards. On average, most symptoms last around four years from the last period. However, around 1 in every 10 women experiences them for up to 12 years and they can be prevented by HRT.

As with men, it's a good time to assess your health and decide how you want to keep it at an optimal level for the second half of your life. Apart from the stock-taking involved in an assessment of your medical history, and filling in questionnaires about your present health and blood tests, mammography, cervical cytology and some bone densitometry would be a good idea. Don't expect your insurance company or the NHS to pay for all these as they are not really into preventive medicine or HRT.

It would be an interesting cost–benefit study if some insurance company undertook, even for an additional annual fee to cover the annual cost, carrying out this screening, with or without HRT, and assessed whether it paid for itself by reducing diabetes, diseases related to being over-weight, heart disease and osteoporosis.

The latest American Association of Clinical Endocrinologists (AACE) and American College of Endocrinology (ACE) position statement published in the July issue of *Endocrine Practice* states 'AACE feels it is important to emphasize that one size doesn't fit all when it comes to treating women with menopause', by Rhonda Cobin, MD, past president of AACE and a member of its reproductive endocrinology scientific committee. 'Hormone-replacement therapy [HRT] must be individualized based on a woman's age, time of onset of menopause, and other cardiovascular, metabolic, and genetic factors,' she added.

As some idea of the acceptance of the principles of HRT, the AACE committee notes that no recommendations from its previous guidelines in 2011 have been reversed or changed.

Summary practice points from the British Menopause Society

1. The decision whether to use HRT should be made by each woman having been given sufficient information by her health professional to make a fully informed choice. Unfortunately only a small proportion of general practitioners have undertaken the necessary courses run by bodies such as the British Menopause Society in the UK and North American Menopause Society.
2. The HRT dosage, regimen and duration should be individualised, with annual evaluation of pros and cons.
3. Arbitrary limits should not be placed on the duration of usage of HRT.

The benefits of hormone therapy usually outweigh the risks.

4. HRT prescribed before the age of 60 has a favourable benefit / risk profile – the window of opportunity.
5. It is imperative that women with premature ovarian insufficiency are encouraged to use HRT at least until the average age of the menopause, 50.
6. If HRT is to be used in women over 60 years of age, lower doses should be started, preferably with a transdermal route of administration.
7. It is imperative that in our ageing population research and development of increasingly sophisticated hormonal preparations should continue to maximise benefits and minimise side effects and risks.
8. This will optimise quality of life and facilitate the primary prevention of long term conditions which create a personal, social and economic burden.
9. Use the lowest dose of estrogen which gives you sustained relief of symptoms, but stay on the treatment unless strong indications occur for you to come off it. This last one is controversial, but I think logical. There is no age at which a woman's body takes a vow and stops needing hormones for skin, bones, brain and many other body systems.

Find a good specialist in which you have confidence and become your own specialist in you and have the following routine tests at least once a year:

- Blood tests (they usually come as a routine package)
- Routine screen of kidney and liver function, bone tests (calcium and phosphate), total cholesterol

and HDL cholesterol, hormone tests (estradiol, testosterone, SHBG, LH, FSH.TSH), hematology profile

- Cervical cytology
- Mammography
- Bone densitometry – spine and hips
- Get a genetic profile done for BRAC1 if you have a strong family history of breast cancer. Only 3% of cases have this rare genetic predisposition to breast and ovarian cancer.
- Clinical examination

Start your own health records with review, summary and comments by physician on each visit. Review, with repeat of blood tests and questionnaires at three and six months initially if you start on HRT or any other long-term treatment, and annually as a routine part of the Fifty-Plus Plan. Treat your body like a plant with the regular hormonal watering, not wait till it wilts and then over-water.

Decide how you want to live the second half of your life – the risks you wish to take and those you don't. What is your bucket list and how fit do you need to be and for how long to achieve it? Share decision making with your partner as well as your specialist.

Long-term benefits and risks of hormone replacement therapy

The Figures Vary

The figures quoted in various articles and guidelines relating to the safety of HRT are enough to make your head spin. So-called observational studies, which are derived from the clinical experience of one clinician or group of clinicians, are generally more favourable than those from the so-called placebo-controlled studies usually performed in larger numbers by epidemiologists. The later are regarded as scientifically more pure, but often use not exactly comparable control groups which can completely invalidate the findings of the study.

The figures also show that the risks vary according to the HRT preparation being used and over what period, age, ethnic group, and other risk factors at work in the population.

Also you have to bear in mind that many of the risk factors overlap, for example weight, diabetes and heart disease. Reduce one of these, and you will likely cut down on the others. It's what sales staff call a win-win situation. Many of the effects of testosterone and estrogens also have overlapping benefits.

Finally, a cynical researcher once said that statistics will confess to anything if you torture them long enough, so many studies will come to different conclusions according to their authors' clinical viewpoint.

Let's now consider the risks in relation to the naturally occurring frequency of the disease.

Causes of death in women over 50:

1. Heart Disease – (10.1 % of deaths over 50 in both UK and US)

Though not generally recognised, the biggest cause of death in women over 50 is heart disease. It about twice as many as die of breast cancer. Therefore women should consider their heart attack risks first when deciding on HRT and minimising it by giving up smoking.

When estrogen-only preparations are concerned the figures are remarkably favourable, giving a 40–50% reduction in cardiovascular events in most clinical studies. When you add in progestins the figures become less favorable, but it does not become actively hazardous.

The reassuring message from NICE (National Institute for Clinical Excellence in the UK) is

1. Ensure that menopausal women and healthcare professionals involved in their care understand that HRT:
    - does not increase cardiovascular disease risk when started in women aged under 60 years
    - does not affect the risk of dying from cardiovascular disease.
2. Be aware that the presence of cardiovascular risk factors is not a contraindication to HRT as long as they are optimally managed.
3. Explain to women that:
    - the baseline risk of coronary heart disease and stroke for women around menopausal age varies from one woman to another according to the presence of cardiovascular risk factors.
    - HRT with oestrogen alone is associated with no, or reduced, risk of coronary heart disease.
    - HRT with oestrogen and progestogen is associated with little or no increase in the risk of coronary heart disease.

2. Breast Cancer (10% of deaths over 50 in both US and UK)

This is the one uppermost in most women's minds when considering HRT. The risks have been well summarised for 1,000 women aged 50–59 by an off-shoot of the British Menopause Society called Women's Health Concern.

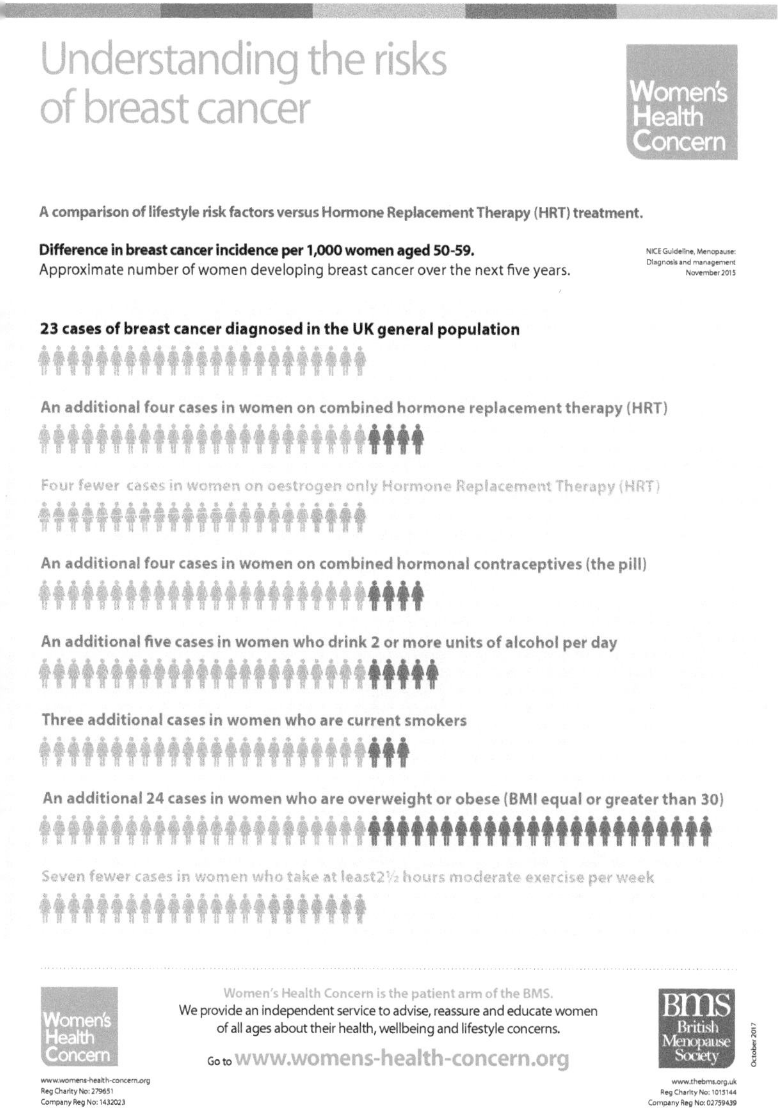
Understanding the risks of breast cancer

Women's Health Concern

A comparison of lifestyle risk factors versus Hormone Replacement Therapy (HRT) treatment.

Difference in breast cancer incidence per 1,000 women aged 50-59.
Approximate number of women developing breast cancer over the next five years.

NICE Guideline, Menopause: Diagnosis and management November 2015

23 cases of breast cancer diagnosed in the UK general population

An additional four cases in women on combined hormone replacement therapy (HRT)

Four fewer cases in women on oestrogen only Hormone Replacement Therapy (HRT)

An additional four cases in women on combined hormonal contraceptives (the pill)

An additional five cases in women who drink 2 or more units of alcohol per day

Three additional cases in women who are current smokers

An additional 24 cases in women who are overweight or obese (BMI equal or greater than 30)

Seven fewer cases in women who take at least2½ hours moderate exercise per week

Women's Health Concern

www.womens-health-concern.org
Reg Charity No: 279651
Company Reg No: 1432023

Women's Health Concern is the patient arm of the BMS.
We provide an independent service to advise, reassure and educate women of all ages about their health, wellbeing and lifestyle concerns.

Go to www.womens-health-concern.org

BMS British Menopause Society

www.thebms.org.uk
Reg Charity No: 1015144
Company Reg No: 02759439

October 2017

This simple figure illustrates that factors in your lifestyle can affect your chances of getting breast cancer far more than whether or not you take HRT. Keeping your weight within the normal range, for example, and taking some exercise, will counteract any effect of starting HRT, as well as lessening your risks of developing heart trouble or diabetes.

Also with modern treatments, especially when caught at an early stage, the 5-year survival from breast cancer is 80%. The secret of early diagnosis is checking for lumps at monthly intervals, and ultrasound or mammography at yearly intervals.

You may be able to get on low risk estrogen-only treatment after a few years on combined estrogen and progestogen treatment, or a preparation called Tibolone which combines the benefits of the two together, sometimes enhancing desire. Take the other risk factors into account before making your decision as illustrated at the end of this section.

3. Stroke

NICE's advice:

1. Explain to women that taking oral (but not transdermal) oestrogen is associated with a small increase in the risk of stroke. Also explain that the baseline population risk of stroke in women aged under 60 years is very low.

Compared to white women, African-American women have more strokes and have a higher risk of disability and death from stroke. This is partly because more African-American women have high blood pressure, a major stroke risk factor. Women who smoke or who have high blood pressure, atrial fibrillation (a kind of irregular heart beat), heart disease, or diabetes are more likely to have a stroke. Hormonal changes with pregnancy, childbirth, and menopause are also linked to an increased risk of stroke.

4. Venous Thromboembolism

NICE's advice:

1. Explain to women that:
   - The risk of venous thromboembolism (VTE) is increased by oral HRT compared with baseline population risk
   - The risk of VTE associated with HRT is greater for oral than transdermal preparations
   - The risk associated with transdermal HRT given at standard therapeutic doses is no greater than baseline population risk.
2. Consider transdermal rather than oral HRT for menopausal women who are at increased risk of VTE, including those with a BMI over 30 kg/m.
3. Consider referring menopausal women at high risk of VTE (for example, those with a strong family history of VTE or a hereditary thrombophilia) to a haematologist for assessment before considering HRT.
4. Absolute rates of stroke vary for different types of HRT compared with no HRT (or placebo), different durations of HRT use and time since stopping HRT for menopausal women.

5. Type 2 Diabetes

NICE's advice:

1. Explain to women that taking HRT (either orally or transdermally) is not associated with an increased risk of developing type 2 diabetes.

2. Ensure that women with type 2 diabetes and all healthcare professionals involved in their care are aware that HRT is not generally associated with an adverse effect on blood glucose control.
3. Consider HRT for menopausal symptoms in women with type 2 diabetes after taking comorbidities into account and seeking specialist advice if needed.

6. Osteoporosis

This is the big area of benefit of HRT, particularly in relation to fragility fractures, which are a type of pathologic fracture that occurs as result of normal activities, such as a fall from standing height or less. There are three fracture sites said to be typical of fragility fractures: vertebral fractures, fractures of the neck of the femur, and Colles fracture of the wrist. The benefits of reducing the osteoporosis which causes this type of fracture should be weighed against all the other far less frequent side-effects of HRT.

Hip fractures are routinely disabling and in 30% of women can be fatal. Added to this are vertebral fractures and gradual vertebral collapse. These are painful and disabling and cause loss of height. The bowing of the back due to these is called 'Dowager's hump'. Losing bone is a normal part of the ageing process, but some people lose bone density much faster than normal. This can lead to osteoporosis and an increased risk of fractures.

Women also lose bone rapidly in the first few years after the menopause, another reason for starting HRT as soon as symptoms appear. Women are more at risk of osteoporosis than men, particularly if the menopause begins early (before the age of 45).

Hip fracture is a very common injury mainly affecting

older people. It is one of the most common reasons for being admitted to a bone (orthopaedic) treatment ward in a hospital. Around 75,000 hip fractures are treated each year in the UK. However, given the UK's ageing population, this number is predicted to double by 2050.

About 8 in 10 people who fracture a hip are women. The average age of someone who fractures their hip is 80 years.

'Nearly all women would trade off almost their entire life expectancy to avoid the state of being admitted to a nursing home', Salkeld and colleagues write. 'Eighty percent of respondents said they would rather be dead'. The authors say comments made during the interviews suggest that fears about what can happen after a hip fracture are based on experiences of parents, friends, and siblings as well as the poor outcomes of hip fracture reported in the medical literature. Studies show that approximately 20% of elderly people who fracture a hip die within one year, and many who do recover need assistance with everyday activities.

Other risk factors include:

- long-term use of high-dose oral corticosteroids
- other medical conditions – such as inflammatory conditions, hormone-related conditions, or malabsorption problems
- a family history of osteoporosis – particularly history of a hip fracture in a parent
- long-term use of certain medications which can affect bone strength or hormone levels
- having a low body mass index (BMI)
- heavy drinking and smoking
- HRT usually prevents osteoporosis, which can be detected early by bone densitometry (DEXA scanning). This is a quick safe and painless procedure, only taking 5–10 minutes.

NICE's advice:

1. Give women advice on bone health and discuss these issues at review appointments
2. Explain to women that the baseline population risk of fragility fracture for women around menopausal age in the UK is low and varies from one woman to another
3. Explain to women that their risk of fragility fracture is decreased while taking HRT and that this benefit:
    - is maintained during treatment but decreases once treatment stops
    - may continue for longer in women who take HRT for a greater time.

Other groups who are at risk of developing osteoporosis include:

- people who have been taking steroid medication for more than three months
- women who have had their ovaries removed
- people with a family history of osteoporosis
- people with an eating disorder such as anorexia or bulaemia.
- people who don't exercise regularly
- people who smoke or drink heavily

I sometimes get the image of little, bent old ladies (Hell's Grannies), battering to death with their umbrellas the doctors who denied them HRT and committed them to years of pain and deformity.

The psychological effects of estrogen deficiency start earlier than other symptoms including the hot flushes and night sweats, and are worse with stress.

NICE's advice:

- There is limited evidence suggesting that HRT may improve muscle mass and strength
- This is important for activities of daily living, and preventing osteoporosis, together with maintaining posture and gait.

The window of opportunity

This is the first five to ten years after hormones hit the floor as your ovaries pack up. It is important for two reasons. Firstly because that's the time when the damage to your physical and mental health starts, especially in the heart, bones and brain.

Secondly, that's when its safest to start HRT, especially as far as both breast cancer and heart disease are concerned. So let's look out of that window and make the decision early on and decide whether HRT is for you.

Often this opportunity of getting maximum benefit for minimum risk is lost because of not recognizing the symptoms of the menopause, ignoring them because you can't have reached that age yet, hope they will go away, or that your friends and even medical advisors have said you should tough it out for as long as possible and not make a fuss.

You should make a fuss and take the decision at or soon after the menopause about whether you want to start on HRT. It's important to detect by the characteristic symptoms when your estrogen levels are dropping and your entering the menopause because much of its impact on your health happens in the first couple of years. It's like watering a plant – leave it to too long and it wilts, often permanently!

Skin condition

A woman's skin needs estrogen to stay in good condition

and only age slowly. While this can be supplied by topical application, the amount needed is very uncertain and can be patchy, so it is much better supplied by HRT. It also prevents dry vagina on intercourse and helps maintain enjoyment of sexual activity by both partners. HRT also helps lubrication and maintains enjoyment of intercourse. These physical factors also help keep sex enjoyable for both partners.

Post menopausal depression is quite common and often severe. It has led to the break-up of many a marriage, especially when accompanied by a drop in libido for both partners and erectile dysfunction. It is often worse when accompanied by hot flushes and night sweats, especially if these are accompanied by loss of sleep. Often these psychological problems start earlier than other symptoms, including the hot flushes, and night sweats become worse with stress.

Memory and mood disorders become worse with the menopause and are best avoided by starting HRT during the early critical period. Why wait until they are established and more difficult to shift?

Memory and mood disorders become worse with the menopause and are best avoided by starting HRT during the early critical period. Why wait until they are established and difficult if not impossible to shift?

Prof RD Langer has written two important papers on the benefits and safety of HRT, the first in 2012, the second in 2017.

In the years since the first WHI report, we have learned much about the characteristics of women who are likely to benefit from HRT. The range of HRT regimens has also increased. Not all women have indications for HRT, but for those who do and who initiate within 10 years of menopause, benefits are both short-term (vasomotor, and avoiding dyspareunia), and long-term (bone health, coronary risk reduction). Critically, the 'facts' that most women and clinicians consider in making the decision to use, or not use, HRT are frequently wrong or incorrectly applied.

Views of the benefits and risks of HRT changed dramatically in 2002 with the unexpected early termination of the CEE + MPA trial and the alarming initial WHI report. HRT use plummeted world-wide by up to 80%, driven by fear of breast cancer and scepticism about cardiovascular benefits.

Over recent years, reanalysis of the data and consideration of further research has led to a better understanding of risk. The overall recognition is that for most women who commence HRT under the age of 60, or within 10 years of the menopause, HRT provides more benefits than risks. The benefits have already been summarized.

To add further evidence to support this view, Professor Robert D Langer describes the process which led to the WHI publication in *JAMA* in July 2002, and explains the true findings of WHI. He reveals that the study did not show any statistically significant increased risk of breast cancer or heart disease in women using HRT, yet the highly publicized conclusions emphasized these risks. Furthermore, the study was designed to test the effects of HRT in older women only, yet the conclusions applied the exaggerated risks to all women.

Published online in *Climacteric*, the journal of the International Menopause Society, this important revelation must surely put the incorrect perception of risks of HRT from WHI to rest and must also call into question the publication process.

Not every woman requires HRT, but all should have access to accurate information about consequences of menopause and treatment options and the reassurance that HRT remains a low risk, beneficial treatment for most women.

Stunningly, the contrasting findings of the WHI trial of CEE alone reported two years later – suggesting prevention of coronary heart disease in women who began HRT at age <60 years, and a reduction in breast cancer overall – were largely ignored. Key lessons from the WHI are that the effects of HRT on most organ systems vary by age and time since last physiologic exposure to hormones and that there are differences between regimens.

Finally, there is very reassuring news from the latest studies reported by the North American Menopause Society where the Chair of their 20 member advisory panel, JoAnn Pinkerton MD, according to an article in October 2017 called has written an article 'Changing the conversation about hormone therapy in menopause'.

In their Journal Menopause, Dr Pinketon emphasizes "We really want clinicians to change the conversation with women. We want them to feel very comfortable that if a woman is having bothersome menopausal systems – hot flashes, night sweats, sleep disturbances – hormone therapy is safe and effective, primarily for women who are starting hormone therapy if they are under 60 and within 10 years of menopause, where there are more benefits than risks."

Dr Pinkerton emphasized the differences in risk between estrogen therapy and estrogen with progestin. Estrogen-only therapy, for example, appears to have a better safety profile for longer use. She emphasized that fear had been driving the conversation about hormone therapy. **"The pendulum is swinging back in favor of hormone therapy"**.

The risk–benefit profile is not static, but in general the balance of benefits and risks for HRT is most favorable when started in the window of opportunity in the first 10 years after menopause, which is known as the timing hypothesis. Choose whether to fly through the 'Window of Opportunity'!

I suggest you find a gynecologist or clinic specializing in HRT and consider pros and cons.

The next chapter has ideas for helping you contact private medical practitioners and guiding you to web sites in both UK and USA willing to provide TRT and HRT advice.

Chapter 4 – The Fifty-Plus Plan

As explained before, for both men and women, generally around the age of fifty, as soon as andropausal or menopausal symptoms begin, there is a window of safety and maximum benefit for starting hormone treatments.

Finding a doctor able and willing to prescribe the hormone replacement therapy is not likely to be easy, in either the US or UK. I am trying to make this easier in both countries, and indeed around the world by putting together like-minded doctors via a web-site www.hormonalhealthcare.co.uk which hopefully will provide a network of doctors who can provide HRT for either men or women, or both, with advice and long-term treatment. You could call them mediatricians – a new specialty is born!

With the help of the medical advisor of your choice, seize the day and seek their opinion on whether you would benefit from starting and continuing treatment. If so, the transdermal route of treatment appears the safest and most economic especially if 'bioidentical' preparations are used such as ethinylestradiol and testosterone.

After the initial assessment, a follow-up visit 3–4 months into treatment is usually required to assess your response to the treatment, relief of symptoms and generally how it affects your quality of life being the most important factors. It you feel the treatment is overall beneficial and you wish to continue, then six-monthly or yearly follow up is usually sufficient unless there are chronic conditions such as diabetes or hypertension to be managed.

Assume that you are on HRT or TRT for life unless you develop a condition develops which is directly related to the treatment, and do not assume you should come off just because you have been on it a set number of years.

At this stage you will have gathered that the Fifty-Plus Plan is that around the age of fifty both men and women should, with the help of a physician with a special interest in hormone replacement treatment, undertake a review of their health, and make a plan for maintaining or even improving it in the second half of their lives. Like going to an accountant to find out how your personal health account is doing.

I hope by now I have been able to overcome the objections that many doctors will raise to the idea of their patients starting hormones on a preventive medical basis. However if you don't look after your health after the age of fifty, it won't look after you. It's time for a stock taking. What illnesses have you had in the past or have at present which might affect your future health? What steps do you need to take to minimize their impact? Without going on a guilt trip or reducing the pleasures in life, what lifestyle factors such as over-eating, smoking, drinking or lack of exercise could you change to help you maintain good health? How well are you at present and what illnesses, if any, need treating?

Conclusions

I hope to have been able to show you how hormonal treatments can enable extension of healthy lives for both men and women from fifty to eighty and well beyond. It can become the basis for a regular six-monthly or yearly health review assessing the strengths and weakness of that person's lifestyle, and correcting that where possible, and looking out for any hormone related problems. These 'hormonal healthcare' clinics could be run by gynecologists, andrologists or general physicians, preferably in their fifties to eighties themselves to get a mature viewpoint of the ageing process and the inevitability of death at the right time.

Current medical thought is that after trying all other non-hormonal treatments for the often severe and even life-wrecking symptoms which usually occur around the age of fifty, men, if they have the characteristic symptoms of the 'andropause', and women if their periods have ceased and they want it, can try hormonal treatment. Usually it is suggested to both sexes that if it is tried at all, even if the results are excellent, they should only try it for a year or two, and then for the shortest possible time. However, given the many benefits of the hormonal treatments to both sexes, and the low level of proven harm – see references – why not keep going?

If there is a comparison with how you treat your car: you get your car serviced every six months or year at most. Why don't you give your body the same regular attention even if it costs a similar amount?

Many patients born with impaired testicular function have been kept in good health for over fifty years with testosterone pellet implants. When men ask me when they should come off testosterone, I tend to answer them, with all due seriousness, only after fifty years, and I mean it! Oh, and the same for HRT with estrogens!

Other Books by Professor Carruthers

1. *The Western Way of Death: Stress, Tension and Heart Disease*, 1973
2. *Fats on Trial*, 1975
3. *Real Health: The Ill Effects of Stress and Their Prevention*, 1980
4. *F/40: Fitness on Forty Minutes a Week*, 1978
5. *Male Menopause: Restoring Vitality and Virility*, 1996
6. *Maximising Manhood: Beating the Male Menopause*, 1997
7. *The Testosterone Revolution: Rediscover Your Energy and Overcome the Symptoms of the Male Menopause*, 2001
8. *ADAM: Androgen Deficiency in the Adult Male – Causes, Diagnosis, and Treatment*, 2004
9. *Testosterone Resistance: Fighting for the men's health Hormone*, 2016
10. *ADAM Androgen Deficiency in the Adult Male – Causes, Diagnosis, and Treatment*, Second Edition 2016.

Published Papers by Professor Carruthers on Testosterone (Refereed)

1. M. Carruthers, 'HRT for the Aging Male: A Clinical Study in 1,000 Men', *The Aging Male*, 1/1 (1998), 34.
2. M. Carruthers, 'Androgen Deficiency in the Aging Male (ADAM): A Multilevel and Multinational Crisis', *The Aging Male*, 14/3 (2000), 58.
3. M. Carruthers, 'More Effective Testosterone Treatment: Combination with Sildenafil and Danazol', *The Aging Male*, 3/1 (2000), 16.
4. M. Carruthers, 'A Multifactorial Approach to Understanding Andropause', *Journal of Sexual and Reproductive Medicine*, 1/2 (2001), 69–74.
5. M. Carruthers, 'The Safety of Long-Term Testosterone Treatment', *The Aging Male*, 4/4 (2002), 255.
6. M. Carruthers, 'The Diagnosis of Androgen Deficiency', *The Aging Male*, 4/4 (2002), 254.
7. M. Carruthers, 'Androgens and the Blood/Brain Barrier', *Andrologia*, 36/3 (2004), 212–213.
8. M. Carruthers and T. R. Trinick, 'The Validity of Androgen Assays', *The Aging Male*, 10/3 (2004), 165.
9. M. R. Feneley and M. Carruther, 'PSA Monitoring during Testosterone Replacement Therapy: Low Long-Term Risk of Prostate Cancer with Improved Opportunity for Cure', *Andrologia*, 36/4 (2004), 212.
10. K. A. Bates, A. R. Harvey, M. Carruthers, and R. N. Martins, 'Androgens, Andropause and Neurodegeneration: Exploring the Link between

Steroidogenesis, Androgens and Alzheimer's Disease', *Cellular and Molecular Life Sciences*, 62/3 (2005), 281–292.
11. M. Carruthers, 'Transdermal Testosterone Treatments', *JEAMM*, 1/2 (2005), 24–27.
12. M. Carruthers, 'An Androgen Resistance Syndrome (ARS) in the Adult Male?', *The Aging Male*, 9/1 (2006), 5.
13. M. R. Feneley and M. E. Carruthers, 'Androgens: The Prostate and Safety of Testosterone Treatment', *The Aging Male*, 9/1 (2006), 4.
14. M. Carruthers, T. R. Trinick, and M. J. Wheeler, 'The Validity of Androgen Assays', *The Aging Male*, 10/3 (2007), 165–172.
15. M. Carruthers, 'The Paradox Dividing Testosterone Deficiency Symptoms and Androgen Assays: A Closer Look at the Cellular and Molecular Mechanisms of Androgen Action', *Journal of Sexual Medicine*, 5/4 (2008), 998–1,012.
16. M. Carruthers, T. R. Trinick, E. Jankowska, and A. M. Traish, 'Are the Adverse Effects of Glitazones Linked to Induced Testosterone Deficiency?', *Cardiovascular Diabetology*, 7 (2008), 30.
17. E. J. Wahjoepramono, L. K. Wijaya, K. Taddei, G. Martins, M. Howard, R. K. de, et al., 'Distinct Effects of Testosterone on Plasma and Cerebrospinal Fluid Amyloid-Beta Levels', *Journal of Alzheimer's Disease*, 15/1 (2008), 129–137.
18. M. Carruthers, 'Time for International Action on Treating Testosterone Deficiency Syndrome', *The Aging Male*, 12/1 (2009), 21–28.
19. M. Carruthers and M. R. Feneley, 'Endocrine

Changes in Different Forms of Long-Term Testosterone Treatment: The UK Androgen Study (UKAS)', *Journal of Sexual Medicine* (2011).
20. M. Carruthers, 'Sex Steroids and Alzheimer's Disease (invited paper)', *Journal of Aging Research* (2011).
21. M. Carruthers, 'The Concept of Androgen Resistance in the Testosterone Deficiency Syndrome', *Journal of Reproductive Medicine and Endocrinology*, 8/3 (2011), 201–202.
22. M. R. Feneley and M. Carruthers, 'Is Testosterone Treatment Good for the Prostate? Study of Safety During Long-Term Treatment', *Journal of Reproductive Medicine and Endocrinology*, 8/3 (2011), 206.
23. T. R. Trinick, M. R. Feneley, H. Welford, and M. Carruthers, 'International Web Survey Shows High Prevalence of Symptomatic Testosterone Deficiency in Men', *The Aging Male*, 14/1 (2011), 10–15.
24. M. Carruthers, 'Testosterone Deficiency Syndrome: Cellular and Molecular Mechanism of Action', *Current Aging Science*, 6/1 (2013), 115–124.
25. R. Martins and M. Carruthers, 'Testosterone as the Missing Link between Pesticides, Alzheimer's Disease, and Parkinson's Disease', *JAMA Neurology*, 71/9 (2014), 1,189–1,190.
26. P. R. Asih, E. J. Wahjoepramono, V. Aniwiyanti, L. K. Wijaya, K. De Ruyck, K. Taddei, et al., 'Testosterone Replacement Therapy in Older Male Subjective Memory Complainers: Double-Blind Randomized Crossover Placebo-Controlled

Clinical Trial of Physiological Assessment and Safety', *CNS and Neurological Disorders – Drug Targets*, 14/5 (2015), 576–586.
27. M. Carruthers, P. J. Cathcart, and M. R. Feneley, 'Evolution of Testosterone Treatment over 25 Years: Symptom Responses, Endocrine Profiles and Cardiovascular Changes', *The Aging Male*, 18/4 (2015), 217–227.

Summary of Testosterone Resistance: The Fight for the Male Hormone

This is a controversial account of why, because of the barriers to testosterone action in the body, men can have normal levels of testosterone but still have life-, love-, and health-wrecking symptoms of testosterone deficiency which need treatment.

The deficiency is increasingly being linked to common and serious medical conditions such as obesity, diabetes, heart and circulatory disorders, and even Alzheimer's disease. This has clearly been shown by the author's pioneering research publications as well as those of other colleagues and researchers worldwide.

However, in the majority of cases, they are often denied this because of the lack of understanding of the medical profession and other authorities regulating the treatment.

This is a wake-up call to both doctors and patients alike to treat the symptoms of testosterone deficiency and related conditions with what the author argues is the most effective, safest, and economic form of preventive medicine of the twenty-first century.

About the Author

Founder and chief medical consultant to the Centre for Men's Health, Professor Malcolm Carruthers is a highly respected men's health specialist and world authority on testosterone deficiency. Dr Carruthers is adjunct professor at the Alzheimer's and Aging Department, Edith Cowan University, Western Australia.

As well as being a fellow of the Royal College of Pathologists, he is a life member of the Royal College of General Practitioners (RCGP). He is also president of the Society for the Study of Androgen Deficiency (Andropause Society), a member of the British Cardiovascular Society, the European Academy of Andrology, the International and European Societies for the Study of the Aging Male, and a past president of the Society for Psychosomatic Research.

Alongside over 120 refereed papers in medical journals and editorials in the *American Heart Journal* and *The Lancet*, he is the author of eight other books including *The Testosterone Revolution* (published by Thorson's/ HarperCollins in 2001) and *ADAM: Androgen Deficiency in the Adult Male – Causes, Diagnosis, and Treatment*, published by Taylor & Francis in 2004, with a second edition printed by Xlibris in 2017. He also published a book describing the new theory of resistance to testosterone being the case of reduced activity rather than reduced amounts of the hormone with Authorhouse in 2017.

Lightning Source UK Ltd.
Milton Keynes UK
UKHW02f1237280618
324920UK00009B/160/P

9 781912 262946